AF397643

The Relevance of
Ethnic Factors
in the
Clinical Evaluation of Medicines

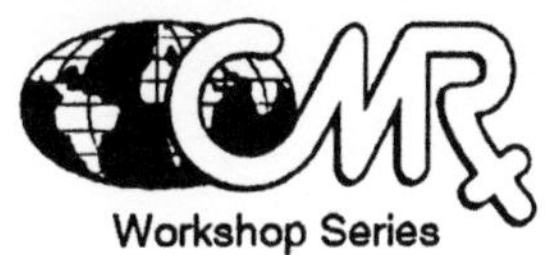

The Relevance of
Ethnic Factors
in the
Clinical Evaluation of
Medicines

Edited by

Stuart Walker
Director

Cyndy Lumley
Associate Director

Neil McAuslane
Project Manager

Centre for Medicines Research
Carshalton, Surrey, UK

Proceedings of a Workshop held at The Medical Society
of London, UK, 7th and 8th July, 1993

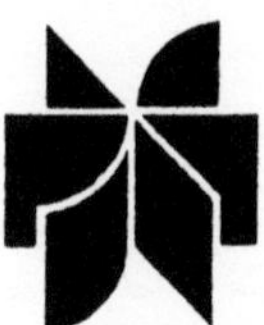

SPRINGER-SCIENCE+BUSINESS MEDIA, B.V.

A catalogue record for this book is available from the British Library

ISBN 978-94-010-4621-3

Library of Congress Cataloging-in-Publication Data

The relevance of ethnic factors in the clinical evaluation of medicines /
  edited by Stuart Walker, Cyndy Lumley, Neil McAuslane.
      p.   cm. — (CMR workshop series)
    "Centre for Medicines Research, Carshalton, Surrey, UK."
    Includes bibliographical references and index.
    ISBN 978-94-010-4621-3   ISBN 978-94-011-1420-2 (eBook)
    DOI 10.1007/978-94-011-1420-2
    1. Drugs—Prescribing—Cross-cultural studies—Congresses.
  2. Ethnic groups—Congresses. I. Walker, Stuart R., 1944–
  II. Lumley, C.E. (Cyndy E.) III. McAuslane, J.A. Neil.
  IV. Centre for Medicines Research (Surrey, England) V. Series.
    [DNLM: 1. Clinical Trials—congresses. 2. Drug Evaluation—
  congresses 3. Ethnic Groups—congresses. QV 771 R382 1994]
  RM138.R45   1994
  615. ´ . 1901—dc20
  DNLM/DLC
  for Library of Congress   94-1681
                                                                CIP

Lasertypeset by Martin Lister Publishing Services, Bolton-le-Sands,
Carnforth, Lancs.

Contents

Contents

Preface

For a research-based pharmaceutical company to be successful in the 1990s, it must have a strategic plan for the global development of new chemical entities. Global development can be defined as an attempt to reach all major markets as rapidly as possible and for many companies these will include the United States, Japan, Germany, France, Italy, UK and Canada, which together represent approximately 85% of the pharmaceutical market in the developed world. The mutual acceptance of foreign clinical data would reduce the time and resources required to develop a new medicine for the international market by eliminating the requirement for the routine repetition of clinical studies in local populations. In Japan this has been largely based on the belief that genetic differences in responsiveness may result in a different benefit/risk assessment for a new medicine, while requests in Europe and the United States for local data relate mainly to methodological and cultural considerations. The importance of this issue has been recognised internationally as it was one of the topics discussed at the International Conference on Harmonisation in Orlando (October 1993) and it is currently on the programme for ICH3 which will be convened in Yokohama in Japan in November 1995.

At the tenth CMR Workshop, an invited group of experts representing academia, regulatory agencies and the pharmaceutical industry from Japan, North America and Europe met for two days to address the issues surrounding the problem of ethnic factors in the clinical evaluation of medicines. The objectives were to review the current situation, address the scientific basis for repeating clinical trials in different ethnic groups and to assess the relevance of inter-ethnic and environmental differences in responsiveness for drug development. During the two days, a variety of topics was debated, ranging from a full and frank discussion on genetic polymorphism in drug metabolism and the consequences, to the clinical implications in both ADME studies and dose-response investigations. Of particular interest was a presentation by Professor Naito which critiqued the current evaluation methods for clinical trials of drugs in Japan, examining the basis of efficacy, safety and utility assessments which may well be one of the major reasons for the observed ethnic differences between Japan and Western countries. Current approaches to global medicines development were reviewed, both from a European and Japanese perspective. The acceptability of foreign data in the registration of new medicines was commented on by various regulatory participants and, following a presentation on the CMR survey on inter-ethnic differences in clinical responsiveness, the implications of these investigations for the design and interpretation of Phase III pivotal studies was debated.

From this meeting, it would seem that inter-ethnic differences based on pharmacogenetics alone should not be a hindrance to the mutual acceptance of foreign clinical data. This CMR Workshop provided an ideal forum for these issues to be debated and a number of important questions were raised during the final discussion session. Because of the importance of this topic, the proceedings of the Workshop have been published so that a wider audience would have the opportunity of reviewing the issues that are so critical to efficient drug development.

The Workshop would not have been possible if we had not been fortunate enough to have some of the leading experts on this topic who gave such excellent presentations. The organisation of the meeting was the responsibility of Dr Christine Harvey, Research Associate at the Centre, and the excellent secretarial support for the meeting was provided by Iris D'Souza. The Editors would like to express their sincere appreciation to both Christine and Iris for organising this meeting so well. However, the majority of work necessary to produce the Workshop proceedings has fallen on the shoulders of Sandra Cox who produced the desktop version of the manuscripts, liaised with the authors and was the main contact with Kluwer. Without Sandra's commitment, observance of deadlines and attention to detail, this volume would not have been produced on time.

Stuart Walker
Cyndy Lumley
Neil McAuslane
April 1994

Notes on Contributors

Luc P Balant PhD is Reader in Pharmacotherapy at the Faculty of Medicine, University of Geneva. He graduated in chemistry from the University of Basle and went on to obtain his doctorate at the Institute of Clinical Biochemistry of the Faculty of Medicines of Geneva. For ten years, he was responsible for the Clinical Pharmacokinetics Laboratory of the Department of Medicine in Geneva, during which time he took sabbatical leave at the Schools of Pharmacy, University of Florida in Gainesville and University of California in San Francisco. He worked for seven years in the pharmaceutical industry as head of Clinical Pharmacology. Since 1987, he has been Head of the Clinical Research Unit at the Psychiatric University Institutions of Geneva. He has written or co-authored more than 300 publications and abstracts, and, over the past 15 years, has sat on the boards of several scientific societies.

Professor Douwe D Breimer PhD is Professor of Pharmacology and Director of Research of the Leiden/Amsterdam Center for Drug Research at Leiden University, and also Chairman of the Center for Human Drug Research at Leiden University Hospital. His research interests are in the areas of drug metabolism, biopharmaceutics and clinical pharmacology (PK/PD inter-relationships). He has (co-)authored over 400 research papers and he is on the editorial boards of 12 international scientific journals. He has received several scientific recognitions, including honorary doctorates from the Semmelweiss University in Budapest, the University of Gent and the University of Uppsala. He is Vice-President of the European Federation for Pharmaceutical Sciences and chairman of ULLA, a European consortium for the advancement of postgraduate pharmaceutical research.

Professor Sir Colin Dollery is the Dean of the Royal Postgraduate Medical School and also the Pro Vice-Chancellor for Medicine and

Dentistry for the University of London. In that capacity he is very much involved with the outcome of the Tomlinson enquiry into London medicine. His research interests are in the action of therapeutic drugs in man and his clinical practice has been mainly in the field of high blood pressure. Sir Colin is the main editor of a two-volume textbook entitled *"Therapeutic Drugs"*. Sir Colin has sat on a number of national committees as a member or chairman, including: the Committee on Safety of Medicines, the Medical Research Council (Chairman of the Physiological Systems Board), The University Grants Committee and Universities Funding Council (Chairman of the Medical Committee).

Lionel D Edwards, MBBS FFPM DObst RCOG is Assistant Vice President, International Clinical Research, Hoffmann-La Roche. He graduated from Guy's Hospital Medical School, London University and worked in family practice, with part-time appointments in Rheumatology and Obstetrics. After seven years of clinical practice, he joined the pharmaceutical industry and over the last 19 years has held various international and US director positions in Clinical Research operations of Roussel, Upjohn, Abbott, and Schering Plough Research Institute. He has been heavily involved in contributing key studies to the FDA and international regulatory authorities on allergy, antibiotic, oncology, cardiovascular and OTC products. He is Chairman of the PMA Special Populations Committee and was the PMA ICH representative for the ICH2 workshop topic "Ethnic Factors in the Acceptability of Foreign Data". Dr Edwards is also a member of the NIH/Institute of Medicine Committee on the Ethical and Legal Issues relating to the Inclusion of Women in Clinical Studies.

Brian A Gennery MB ChB DipPharmMed FFPM is an independent Pharmaceutical Consultant. In this context, one of his main assignments is as the General Manager of the London Liaison Office of the Otsuka Pharmaceutical Company Limited. This office is responsible for carrying out clinical research and development programmes in Europe on original products discovered by the Otsuka Pharmaceutical Company of Japan. Previously, he was Group Medical Director of Europe for Lilly Research Laboratories.He is on the Board of the Faculty of Pharmaceutical Medicine and Deputy Chairman of the British Association of Pharmaceutical Physicians and has been a member of The Association of the British Pharmaceutical Industry (ABPI) Medical Committee. He is on the Editorial Board of *Pharmaceutical Medicine* and has extensive experience in teaching and training, having regular commitments to both the Postgraduate course in Pharmaceutical Medicine of the University of Cardiff, and the MSc in Pharmaceutical Medicine at the University of Surrey.

Professor Charles F George BSc MD FRCP FFPM has been Professor of Clinical Pharmacology, University of Southampton and Honorary Consultant Physician of Southampton and South-West Hants District Health Authority since 1975. He is Dean of the Faculty of Medicine and a Member of the General Medical Council, and is currently Chairman of the Joint Formulary Committee responsible for overseeing the production of the British National Formulary. He is also a member of the Editorial Board of *Adverse Drug Reactions and Poisoning Reviews* and *Journal of Pharmacy and Pharmacology*. His publications include three books, two supplements and more than 150 articles which are mostly in peer-reviewed journals.

Christine Harvey PhD is a management consultant in the London office of Arthur D Little, where she specialises in the healthcare and pharmaceutical industries. She was previously a Senior Research Associate at the Centre for Medicines Research, where her work focused on regulatory issues. Prior to this, she worked in academia and in the biotechnology industry.

John Henderson BSc MB ChB FRCP (Ed) FFPM is Senior Vice President – Medical for the US and International Pharmaceutical Groups of Pfizer Incorporated. Prior to his present appointment he was Executive Vice President for Research and Development for Pfizer Pharmaceuticals in Japan, a position he held for just over two years. Before his transfer to Japan he was Vice President for European Clinical Research and Regulatory Affairs for Pfizer Central Research based in England. His twenty years in the pharmaceutical industry have provided him with a broad-based knowledge of drug development and marketing worldwide.

Kazunori Hirokawa BSc MD PhD graduated from the University of Tokyo and Tokyo Medical and Dental University School of Medicine. After clinical and scientific training he worked as a manager of R&D planning department, Daiichi Pharmaceutical Company Limited. He is a Research Fellow of the Department of Clinical Pharmacology, Royal Postgraduate Medical School, University of London, where he is currently studying clinical trial methodology.

Jean-Marc Husson MD PhD INSEAD/AMP has been Head of Medical Affairs, Pharma Policy Direction, Roussel Uclaf since 1993. During his twenty years in this company, he has run various units involved in Clinical Research and Regulatory Affairs, including the Roussel Uclaf Medical Department. His main activities are now regulatory affairs and quality assurance. Dr Husson is currently Professor at the University of Montpellier I (Pharmaceutical Sciences), and has around 75 publications in international journals, covering animal research, clinical pharmacology and therapeutics in hepatogastroenterology, endocrinology and angiology, as well as regulatory affairs and quality assurance. He is also involved in various official scientific or regulatory committees and learned societies.

Professor Trevor M Jones BPharm PhD FPS CChem FRSC MCPP is Director of Research, Development and Medical, Wellcome Foundation Limited. He is responsible for all R&D and Medical activities worldwide (excluding the USA) and is a Main Board Director. Some time Visiting Professor at the University of North Carolina and the University of Strathclyde, he is currently a Member of Council and Visiting Professor at King's College, London University. Professor Jones is a member of a number of editorial boards and has authored numerous publications throughout his career. He has been a Member of the Medicines Commission (UK Government Department of Health) for twelve years and advises the Cabinet Office on matters relating to the Human Genome Project. He is also an expert on the Task Force on the use of Human Tissues: Nuffield Bioethics Council.

Etienne Labbé graduated in 1975 with honours (Lauréat) from the University of Paris as a Medical Doctor. He then specialised in Clinical Pharmacology, Pharmacokinetics and Statistics at La Pitié-Salpêtrière University Hospital as a post doc. After joining the pharmaceutical industry in 1980, he began working with Japanese researchers and clinical investigators. He is now Medical Director for Japan at Synthelabo and is responsible for Research and Development on the Japanese territory.

Cyndy E Lumley BSc PhD is Associate Director at the Centre for Medicines Research, where she has worked for the past eleven years. Prior to joining the CMR, she obtained a BSc (hons) in Medical Biochemistry from the University of Surrey and a PhD in Radiation Biology from the University of London. Dr. Lumley's current research interests include safety testing of new medicines, drug regulations, the predictive value of animal studies for man, pharmaceutical research and development expenditure, and factors affecting drug development. She is a regular contributor to scientific journals and international meetings, has co-authored over 30 research papers and edited two books.

Neil McAuslane BSc MSc PhD, as Project Manager for the Centre for Medicines Research, is responsible for its safety evaluation/regulations programme. He has degrees in Pharmacology and Toxicology, and joined the Centre to initiate the control animal pathology database project. Dr McAuslane's current research interests involve clinical safety, and the CMR's continuing study into the evaluation of inter-ethnic differences. He has edited two books and co-authored several of the Centre's publications in these research areas.

Professor Chikayuki Naito MD PhD is Professor, The 1st Department of Internal Medicine, School of Medicine, Teikyo University and Honorary Chairman of the Department of Internal Medicine, Tokyo Teishin Hospital. Since 1981, he has served on many Advisory Committees of the MHW: Member of the Standing Committee, Central Pharmaceutical Affairs Council; Chairman of the Subcommittee on New Drugs; Member (1983–1985) and Chairman (1985–1989) of the Committee on Drug Safety, Pharmaceutical Affairs Council. Dr Naito was the Chairman of the three drafting Committees: on General Guidelines for New Drug Approvals; on Statistical Guidelines for New Drug Approvals; and for Guidelines on the Format for New Drug Applications. He was also a Member of the MHW Study Group on Methodology for Phase I Studies and on PMS Studies. He has been a delegate of MHW to ICH in Efficacy from the beginning of ICH and was a rapporteur of the session of "Ethnic Factors in the Acceptability of Foreign Data", and discussant of the session of "Dose Response Information to Support Product Registration" for ICH 2. Dr Naito has authored numerous publications, is a member of many academic committees, and sits on the editorial boards of a number of medical journals. He was President of the Japan Atherosclerosis Society from 1990 to 1992 and was awarded the Ohshima Prize of Japan Atherosclerosis Society in 1991.

Marisa Papaluca MD is Senior Medical Director at the Ministry of Health in Italy, Pharmaceutical Department. After graduation in Medicine in 1978, she completed her residency in internal medicine at the Catholic University in Rome and obtained the relevant

University Certificate in 1983. During her university career she was primarily involved in cellular immunology research and published several scientific papers in that area. In 1984 she joined the Ministry of Health and her main areas of activity focused on the medical evaluation of drugs, in the pharmacovigilance areas as well as for registration procedures. Since 1985 she has been involved in the international harmonisation of scientific regulatory requirements in pharmacovigilance, particularly in the European Union framework. Since 1992 Dr Papaluca has been acting as scientific co-ordinator in Italy for European Concertation Procedures, and she is currently a member of the CPMP Efficacy Working Party and of the E5-ICH Working Group.

John Patterson MB ChB MRCP FFPM is the International Medical Director of Zeneca Pharmaceuticals (formerly ICI), having been their Vice President for Clinical Research and Medical Affairs in the USA and Medical Director of ICI Pharma Germany. He is responsible for all aspects of the human exposure and evaluation of the Company's products. He is a Board Member of the Faculty of Pharmaceutical Medicine and an examiner for the Diploma in Pharmaceutical Medicine. In his 18 years in the pharmaceutical industry he has served on the Medical Committee of The Association of the British Pharmaceutical Industry and numerous other committees and working parties.

Professor Michael D Rawlins BSc MD FRCP FFPM has been Professor of Clinical Pharmacology at the University of Newcastle upon Tyne since 1973. His research interests are in the fields of investigating inter-individual variability in response to drugs, mechanisms of drug toxicity, and pharmacoepidemiology. He is Chairman of the UK Committee on Safety of Medicines.

Professor Jens S Schou MD DSc is Professor of Pharmacology and Toxicology, Department of Pharmacology, Faculty of Medicine, University of Copenhagen, Denmark. He is a member of the Licensing Committee for New Medicines, Chairman of the Adverse Drug Reactions Committee (Danish National Board of Health), and the Pesticide Board (Environmental Protection Agency). Professor Schou's present research is focused on safety testing of pharmaceuticals and pharmacovigilance. He has authored more than 200 publications, ranging from basic pharmacology to pharmacovigilance.

W Leigh Thompson PhD MD received his Doctor of Medicine degree in 1965 from The Johns Hopkins University, where he was a resident for three years on the Osler Medical Service. Dr Thompson joined Eli Lilly and Company in April 1982 as Director of Clinical Investigation and was named an executive director of Lilly Research Laboratories later that year, Vice President in 1986, Group Vice President in 1988, Executive Vice President in January 1992, and Chief Scientific Officer, a newly created position, in February 1993. Dr Thompson is Past President and Honorary Life Member of the Society of Critical Care Medicine and co-editor of *The Textbook of Critical Care Medicine and Critical Care: State of the Art*. He is a Fellow of the American College of Physicians and the American College of Critical Care Medicine, and a member numerous other academic societies.

Katherine Voith holds a Masters degree in Organic Chemistry and a PhD degree in Pharmacology from McGill University in Montreal. For many years, she served as the Head of the CNS Section at Ayerst Research Laboratories where she was responsible for establishing a psychopharmacology research programme that focused upon the development of drugs in the fields of schizophrenia, Parkinson's Disease, Alzheimer's Disease and obesity. She is the author of over 50 publications and holds several patents. In 1984, she joined the Bureau of Human Prescription Drugs which is the Canadian Drug Regulatory Authority. She is also actively involved in ICH-related activities, being the Chairperson of the Canadian expert working group in the area of efficacy.

Professor Stuart R Walker BSc PhD CChem FRSC CBiol FIBiol is the Director of the Centre for Medicines Research in the UK and Honorary Professor of Pharmaceutical Medicine, University of Wales, Cardiff. He spent ten years at London University which included lectureships in biochemical pharmacology at St Mary's Hospital Medical School and in clinical pharmacology at the Cardiothoracic Institute in London. This was followed by eight years with Glaxo Group Research in the UK where he had international responsibility for several of their clinical research programmes. His current research interests include studies into the process of innovation in drug research and development, an examination of the impact of international medicines regulations and policy issues on drug development, investigating the role as well as the predictive value of preclinical animal toxicology and measuring the socioeconomic benefit of medicines in therapeutic intervention studies.

Professor Walker is a member of several academic, professional and industrial committees and sits on the editorial boards of three scientific journals. He is frequently involved in the organisation of national and international meetings on key issues that concern the pharmaceutical industry and has co-authored over 150 research papers and edited thirteen books.

PROBLEMS IN THE ACCEPTABILITY OF FOREIGN CLINICAL DATA FOR PHARMACEUTICALS

1
Acceptability of foreign data: genetic, cultural and environmental differences – do they matter?

LIONEL D EDWARDS

Summary

1. Genetic polymorphism plays an important role in the metabolism of some compounds but age, gender, alcohol, tobacco and diet may also have an impact on the pharmacokinetics of certain products. The significance of these factors however is unclear as much of the literature describes studies using small numbers of patients and volunteers.

2. The situation is further complicated because of differences in culture, nomenclature, diagnosis and medical practice. The latter is illustrated by the US having the objective of curing the patients, in Europe the concern is on management, whereas in Japan the emphasis is on patient comfort so adverse reactions are to be avoided and the lowest effective dose is often selected.

3. In Japan, currently, because of a belief in large differences regarding genetic factors, all clinical work must be repeated in Japanese subjects or patients. In Europe and the United States, data is theoretically interchangeable but a low percentage of studies in practice are mutually acceptable.

Introduction

During the period 1975–1989, the US and Japan lead other developed countries of the world with respect to the number of approved new drugs introduced on to the world market (Barral, 1990) (Figure 1.1). For the US, a major change can be anticipated. This will arise from two major changes in emphasis. Firstly, the US Healthcare Reform Bill has focused attention on the seven cents spent on drugs out of every dollar on health and secondly, until now, the US industry has not had to demonstrate whether the drug was more efficacious than another to gain approval.

Market forces may well achieve in the US what legislation has achieved in Europe and, to a lesser extent, Japan. The number of drugs worldwide in the late stages of investigation (Phase III) may be expected to decline as many are terminated earlier because of efficacy or safety profiles which previously would have been acceptable. This is worrying because many "me too" drugs eventually develop special niches, additional indications or provide more improved patient compliance or convenience than the "gold standard" medicine. Therefore, more money is likely to be spent in the discovery process in the search for novel medicines and, consequently, the later clinical phases will be scrutinised for the cost effectiveness of these medicines. The duplication inherent in clinical global programmes is an obvious target. Currently, the avoidance of duplication is being examined by regulatory authorities and pharmaceutical associations who are now involved in a series of workshops under the auspices of the ICH programme (International Conference on Harmonisation).

Why is clinical data from one region not given automatic regulatory approval and credibility by the other regions? This is because

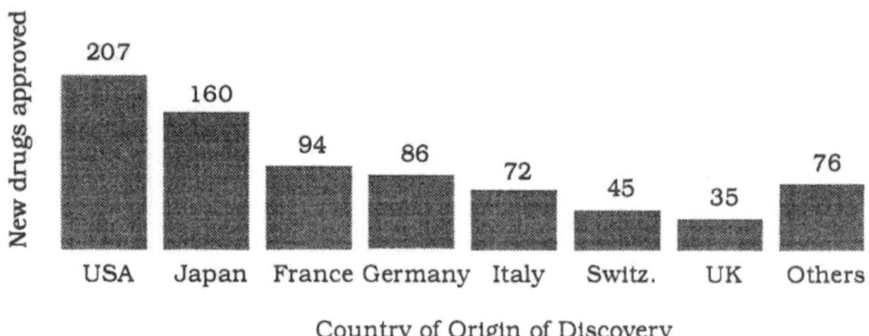

Figure 1.1 New drugs approved 1975–1989. Adapted from Barral (1990)

the administered dosage, common adverse events and even efficacy rates contained within the applications show variations which, even in the absence of a legal requirement, make reviewers want data derived and applicable to their own populations. Differences between nations of 30% or more of adverse events such as nausea and headache do little to reassure both regulatory reviewers and the nations' prescribers without adequate explanation.

Are the differences real? When measured objectively, on occasions they are. More frequently, subjective differences cause most of the variations seen in efficacy and safety which even determine the "optimal dose" of a medicine for a nation irrespective of blood levels, e.g. antibiotics and antihypertensives.

Objective differences

Genetic polymorphism has been described in terms of slow or fast metabolisers with acetylation or oxidative metabolic pathways often involving the family of cytochrome P450 enzymes. Other genetic traits are reported with conjugation pathways, aldehyde dehydrogenase and even with plasma protein binding. Age, gender, alcohol, tobacco, diet and illicit drug use can also have an impact on metabolism. Subsequent papers in this volume will specifically address these issues but the following examples give some idea of the possible racial differences. The acetylation pathway is generally faster in 90% of Japanese, compared to only 45% of the Caucasian and African population. This affects drugs such as isoniazid and clonazepam and caffeine (Wood and Zhou, 1991) (Table 1.1).

Examples of drugs subject to oxidative cytochrome P450 metabolism include metoprolol, propranolol and nifedipine (Wood and Zhou, 1991) (Table 1.2). There are also examples of possible pharmacodynamic differences between races. Wood and Zhou reported that Asians may require smaller doses of neuroleptic drugs and suffer adverse effects at lower doses than Caucasians even after adjustments for body weight. Strickland *et al.* (1991) also reported that with the tricyclic agents, Afro-Americans tend to have high plasma levels, a faster therapeutic effect and more side-effects than Caucasian patients. It is now well recognised that calcium channel blockers or diuretics given as monotherapy for hypertension are more effective in Afro-Americans compared to β-blockers and ACE inhibitors. However, the reverse is true for Caucasians (Hall, 1990; Freis, 1986). Even so, labetalol, a combined α- and β-blocker, can be equally effective in both populations. A final example is the reports of genetic clinical differences with lithium when used for

Table 1.1 Frequency of slow acetylators in some populations

Population	Frequency (%)
Black	
East Africa	55
US	42–51
Caucasian	
Britain	55–62
Germany	57
Canada	59
US	52–58
Chinese	
Hong Kong	22
Taiwan	22
Thailand	34
Mainland China	13
Eskimo	
Canada	5–6
Alaska	21
Japanese	
Japan	7–12
US	10

Adapted from Wood and Zhou (1991).

manic depressive disorders. Asian patients (including the Japanese) are reported to have good therapeutic response at 0.5–0.8 meq/l compared to the levels of US Caucasian patients who require 0.8–1.2 for a good response (Jefferson *et al.*, 1987; Takahashi, 1979).

It is important to note that much of the literature describes studies using small numbers of patients and volunteers and thus the differences could either be real or distorted by a few outliers in the data.

Additional objective ethnic differences

Weight and height leading to differences in fat, muscle and blood volume are responsible for possible variation within a study population, but between racial or ethnic groups this is less obvious. In general, Asians are smaller and leaner than their European or American counterparts, though this is changing, as is the diet in urban Japan. The social use of alcohol and its potentiating effects

Table 1.2 Frequency of poor metabolisers of debrisoquine-type and mephenytoin-type hydroxylation in populations

Population	Frequency (%) Debrisoquine-type	Frequency (%) Mephenytoin-type
American Indian		
Eskimo	—	5—21
Panama	0	—
Arab	1	—
Black		
Ghana	0.7–5	—
Nigeria	3–8	—
Caucasian		
Britain	3–9	—
Germany	5	—
Denmark	7	—
Switzerland	9–10	5.4
Sweden	5.4–8	2.8
Finland	6	—
Hungary	10	—
Spain	6.6–10	—
Canada	7	—
US	7	2.7
Australia	6	—
Chinese		
Canada	31	5.1
China	0–0.7	—
Egyptian	1.4	—
Japanese	0–0.5	18–23

Adapted from Wood and Zhou (1991).

on drug metabolism induction is well known and it may be particularly relevant to abstaining populations (Moslem, Mormon). Finally, reports on differences in diet, additives and salt content and even citrus fruit and how this may alter metabolic rates have been documented (Lin *et al.*, 1988; Henry *et al.*, 1987; Gould *et al.*, 1972; Baily *et al.*, 1991). From this list, it might be supposed that clinical ethnic differences should be more frequently seen, but the reality is that most drugs have such a large benefit to toxic risk ratio, that differences are rarely seen (Edwards, 1992). The drugs that have a sharp dose response for efficacy and safety are usually rejected in the development process or are so valuable that they are developed and only used following individual titration (digoxin, warfarin). Thus ethnic differences are irrelevant for such drugs and not seen unless deliberately sought. A consensus is emerging that real clinical differences due to genetic metabolism and environmental factors are rarer than intra-ethnic variations. The author firmly believes that most variations in clinical response are due to clinical differences in medical practice and culture.

Medical practice, cultural differences and nomenclature

Differences in medical nomenclature and diagnosis are illustrated in Table 1.3

Table 1.3 Examples of differences in nomenclature/diagnosis

USA	*Europe*
Headache	Migraine – France
Migraine	"Liver crisis" – France
Chest pain	Heart pain – Germany
Chronic tiredness or fatigue	Cardiac fatigue – Germany
Anxiety neurosis (variation)	Autonomic dysautonia – UK Vasovegative dystonia – Germany
Appendectomy	Appendicectomy
Lumpectomy (breast lump removal)	Tylectomy – UK
Schizo-affective (older)	Manic. Manic-depressive
Bipolar depression	Hypomania disorders UK, Scandinavia, Germany

Some specific examples of diseases diagnosed in one country but not necessarily identified as a problem elsewhere include:

Postural hypotension or neurovegetative hypotonia only appears to exist in Germany as a condition needing treatment;

British and USA medical practice dismiss coprescription of NSAIDs for respiratory or pelvic infection as scientifically unsound;

Tempero-mandibular joint dysfunction – a US diagnosis;

Spa treatments and liver disorders in France;

Heavy leg syndrome in Switzerland.

Table 1.4 Differences in medical practice

Antibiotics
* West Germany Scrips/Head of Population
      $\frac{1}{2}$ of UK total
      which are
      only $\frac{1}{2}$ of USA total
* Pattern of infectious disease is the same but the willingness to use antibiotics is not

C Section
* USA – Caesarean section is done in over 20% births
  UK   – 7%
  But infant birth mortality is higher in the USA
  Legal and environmental factors influence US practice

There are many differences in medical practice and a few simple examples are shown in Table 1.4 (Payer, 1988). In Japan, polypharmacy is especially valued. Favoured posology can also differ between nations; in the US, rectal suppositories are rarely used but frequently preferred in Continental Europe. In Spain and Italy, the availability of an injectable formula may also be critical to the success of a product. Combination products are welcome in many countries but frowned upon in others.

Probably the most important difference to the three regions of US, Europe and Japan is the *"objective of treatment"*. In the US, the prime objective is to cure the patient. This is pursued with aggressive medication doses with the near to maximum dose being used and if necessary titrated downwards if adverse reactions are poorly tolerated. In Europe, the emphasis is on patient management. This means that doses are titrated up to a mean effective dose compatible with moderate discomfort. In Japan, the emphasis is on patient comfort, so adverse reactions are to be avoided and the lowest effective dose is often selected. As might be expected, these attitudes impact on the observations and judgement of physicians, investigators, patients and reviewers of the data as well as outcome effects.

Patients also respond with ethnic patterns in reporting adverse events. In Japan, it is considered bad form to complain and even worse to complain about gastrointestinal events. Thus nausea, vomiting and bowel events have much lower rates of report in Japan than other nations. None the less, serious adverse events such as gastric bleeding will be reported at similar rates in most nations. From my own experience, Sweden and the USA have very similar rates of reporting for the same drug in clinical studies. Germany, Japan and Switzerland tend to be more stoic about reporting adverse events of a more trivial nature, whereas Italy, France and Britain tend to fall between these two extremes.

Acceptance of foreign data

Twenty years ago, I was told by a UK regulator that English data was very good, Scottish reasonable, Welsh data was acceptable and that US data was not helpful for an English population. This attitude would be unacceptable today though it is recognised that each nation's prescribers may want to see nationally familiar names and universities involved in drug development. In Japan, currently because of their belief of large differences in genetic factors, all clinical work must be repeated in Japanese subjects or patients. In Europe and the US, data is theoretically interchangeable but only 30% of studies are mutually acceptable. The uncertainty of subjective factors, compliance assurance and lack of placebo control are major factors in the US rejection rate. US patient population's relevance to Europe, the high doses used and multiple ethnic European interpretations by reviewers may be factors, though unstated reasons, for European acceptance rates.

The duplication of studies and rejection of data have an impact on the availability of new medicines and the use of investigators', patients', volunteers' and reviewers' time and their goodwill. Clearly, the challenge to academia, industry and the regulatory authorities is to measure the few objective differences when suspected, narrow the subjective influences and develop mutually relevant data measurement methods to account, assess or convert differences into useful global data.

References

Bailey DG, Arnold, JM, Munoz C, Spence JD (1991). Interaction of citrus juices with felodipine and nefidipine. *Lancet*, 337(8736):268–9.

Barral PE (1990). Fifteen years of results of pharmaceutical research in the world. *Perspective et Santé Publique*, 1985 and *Update*, 1990.

Benet L (1992). *Women as Subjects of Research*. Institute of Medicine Workshop, Washington DC.

Edwards LD (1992). Gender and ethnic monitoring. PMA Survey, Reported PERI Workshop.

Freis ED (1986). Antihypertensive agents. In: Kalow W *et al.* (eds) *Ethnic Differences in Reactions to Drugs and Xenobiotics*. Alan R Liss Inc, New York, pp. 313–322.

Gould SE, Hayashi T, Nakashima T, Shohoji T, Tanimura T, Tashiro T (1972). Coronary heart disease and stroke. Atherosclerosis in Japanese Men in Hiroshima, Japan and Honolulu, Hawaii. *Arch Pathol*, **93**(2):98–102.

Hall DH (1990). Pathophysiology of hypertension in blacks. *Am J Hypertens*, **3**:366S–371S.

Henry CJ, Emery B and Piggot S (1987). Basal metabolic rate and diet induced thermogenesis in Asians living in Britain. *Human Nutr Clin Nutr,* **41**(5):397–402.

Jefferson JW, Ackerman DL, Carol JA and Greist JH (1987). *Lithium Encyclopedia for Clinical Practice*. American Psychiatric Press, Washington, DC.

Lin KM, Lesser JM and Poland RE (1986). Ethnicity and psychopharmacology culture. *Med Psychiatry*, **10**:151–65.

Payer L (1988). *Medicine and Culture*. H. Holt, New York.

Strickland TL, Lin KM, Mendoza R, Poland RE, Ranganath V and Smith MW (1991). Psychopharmacologic considerations in the treatment of black American populations. *Psychopharmacol Bull*, **27**(4):441–448.

Takahashi R (1979). Lithium treatment in affective disorders: therapeutic plasma level. *Psychopharmacol Bull*, **15**:32–35.

Wood AJJ and Zhou HH (1989). Ethnic differences in drug disposition and responsiveness. *N Engl J Med*, **320**:565–70.

Wood AJJ and Zhou HH (1991). Ethnic differences in drug disposition and responsiveness. *Clin Pharmacokinet*, **20**:350–373.

2
Genetic polymorphisms in drug metabolism: clinical implications and consequences in ADME studies

DOUWE D BREIMER

Summary

1. Large differences in the metabolism of drugs can exist between different species and within individual populations which may be caused by genetic or environmental factors. For some drugs, the regulation of metabolism is such that the product of a single gene is predominately responsible for mediating a specific pathway. Mutation of the gene results in subpopulations with widely differing abilities to carry out that specific reaction and thus polymorphism is exhibited.

2. Subpopulations can be identified by suitable phenotype procedures directly related to the affected pathway. For example, slow and fast acetylators may be identified by measuring urinary excretion of unchanged versus an acetyleted drug following administration of a sulfonamide. Genetic polymorphisms also exist with respect to drug oxidation and a close relationship has been shown to exist between an individual's ability to oxidise debrisoquine and sparteine and numerous drugs have been identified whose metabolism is affected by this polymorphism (5–10% PM in Caucasian populations but 0–2% in Japanese/Chinese populations). Further work has established genetic polymorphism in drug oxidation with respect to the hydroxylation of S-mephenytoin resulting in poor and fast metabolisers although the number of drugs affected is relatively small. The frequency of the PM phenotype differs according to geographical distribution (Caucasian populations 2–5%, Chinese/Japanese populations 15–23%).

3. Whether or not a deficient pathway in the metabolism of certain drugs has clinical relevance obviously depends on the relative importance of the affected pathway to the overall elimination of the compound. A number of implications are discussed in this paper. Considerable inter-individual variability in drug metabolising activity exists within each phenotypic group. Clinically it should be regarded as equally relevant to detect and distinguish between patients at the extreme ends of unimodal distribution as between patients belonging to the different modes of a bimodal distribution. It is the magnitude rather than the origin of the variability that determines the clinical relevance and therefore there is no fundamental contrast between genetic factors (polymorphism) and environmental factors causing variability in the rate of drug metabolism.

4. Information on a new compound obtained preclinically (e.g. by using human microsomes or enzymes) should be used to optimise Phase I and Phase II clinical studies. Phenotyping is possible either by giving a single probe drug detecting a specific polymorphism or by combining for example sparteine mephenytoin and other probe drugs to obtain a more complete picture of the metabolic status of an individual subject ("cocktail" approach).

Introduction

Large differences have been shown to exist between different species and among different individuals within one species, including man, in their capacity to metabolise drugs and other xenobiotics. This inter-species and inter-individual variability is caused by genetic and environmental factors. The basal rate of drug metabolism in a certain individual is determined by genetic constitution, but it varies in addition with age, gender and environmental factors like diet, disease states, concurrent use of other drugs or exposure to certain xenobiotics (inducing or inhibiting drug metabolising enzyme activity).

During the last 15 years much research interest has been focusing on the genetic factors responsible for variability in the rate of drug metabolism and several recent reviews have been published on this subjects (e.g. Kalow, 1992; Wilkinson, 1989). For many drugs the genetic regulation of their rate of metabolism is polygenic and multifactorial in nature. Multiple and differentially regulated enzymes are involved in the biotransformation process, either with respect to a single metabolic pathway or the overall metabolism of a drug. As a result, the frequency distribution of the drug metabolising activity *in vivo* (intrinsic metabolic clearance) within a human population is continuous or unimodal.

For some drugs, however, monogenic regulation of metabolism has been shown to occur, i.e. the product of a single gene is predominantly responsible for mediating a specific metabolic pathway. Mutations of the gene result in subpopulations with widely differing abilities to carry out that specific metabolic reaction; at the extreme the metabolic activity may be essentially absent. Such mutations may be rare as appears to be the case for the 4′-hydroxylation of phenytoin (Vasko *et al.*, 1980) or they may be more frequent so that polymorphism is exhibited, i.e. the mutations occur in the population more frequently than 1%. Now subpopulations can be identified by suitable phenotype procedures directly related to the affected metabolic pathway. If the latter is a major one in the overall metabolism of a drug, then the overall disposition kinetics of the unchanged drug will also exhibit genetic polymorphism, i.e. bimodality in the frequency distribution of a suitable parameter within a human population. Already 30 years ago this was recognised for the *N*-acetylation of drugs like isoniazid, procainamide, hydralazine, sulfonamides and others. Individual subjects may be phenotyped as rapid or slow acetylators by measuring urinary excretion of unchanged versus acetylated drug. The clinical consequences of this polymorphism have been relatively well established (review: Price Evans, 1992). It is important to note that there are considerable ethnic differences in the frequency of the allele controlling slow acetylation, e.g. in individuals of Caucasian origin the percentage of rapid acetylators varies between 30 and 70%, in Egyptians this is only 10–20%, and in the Japanese population 80–90% (Price Evans, 1992).

In more recent years it has become increasingly clear that genetic polymorphism may also exist with respect to drug oxidation, which is a major route of metabolism for many drugs. In 1977 two groups reported on the discontinuous distribution of the 4'-hydroxylation of the antihypertensive agent debrisoquine in British populations; this was based on the 8 hours' urinary excretion profile of unchanged drug versus 4'-hydroxydebrisoquine (metabolic ratio) (Mahgoub *et al.*, 1977; Tucker *et al.*, 1977). Around the same time separate studies with sparteine in a German population detected a subpopulation of subjects who were deficient in the oxidation of this oxytocic agent (Eichelbaum *et al.*, 1979). In subsequent years a close relationship was shown between an individual's ability to oxidize debrisoquine and sparteine and it is now well established that the two metabolic pathways are regulated by the same genetic alleles. Since then numerous drugs have been identified whose metabolism is in a major or minor way affected by this debrisoquine/sparteine polymorphism (Eichelbaum and Gross, 1992).

In 1984 Küpfer and Preisig reported on another, currently also well established, genetic polymorphism in drug oxidation, i.e. the hydroxylation of S-mephenytoin (Küpfer and Preisig, 1984). The poor metaboliser (PM) phenotype is usually identified by the reduced ability to form and excrete 4'-hydroxymephenytoin in 8 hours' urine. It seems that the number of other drugs whose metabolism is affected by this polymorphic enzyme is relatively small. These include some related anticonvulsant agents (mephobarbital, methylphenytoin), hexobarbital, diazepam and omeprazole (Wilkinson *et al.*, 1992; Andersson *et al.*, 1992; Bertilsson *et al.*, 1989). Interestingly, the frequency of the PM phenotype differs considerably according to geographical distribution, i.e. in Caucasian populations it varies between 2 and 5%, whereas in Chinese and Japanese populations it is as high as 15–23% (Wilkinson *et al.*, 1992).

Because the debrisoquine/sparteine polymorphism co-segregates with the metabolism of many other compounds, this review will further be limited to a brief discussion of the molecular basis, clinical implications and consequences for drug development of this particular genetic polymorphism.

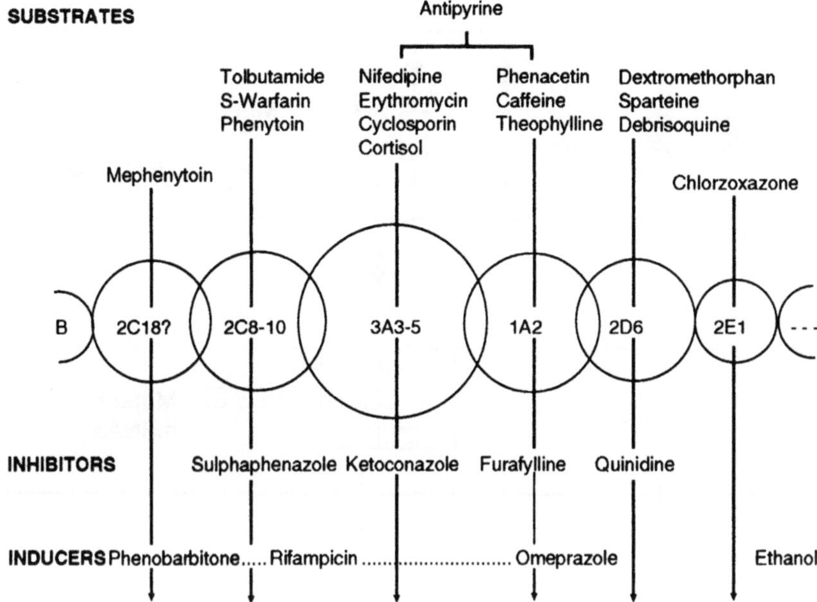

Figure 2.1 Schematic representation of different human cytochromes P-450 enzymes (circles) with their probe substrates, selective inhibitors and inducers (Breimer and Tucker, unpublished; after Breimer, 1983).

Characteristics of the debrisoquine/sparteine polymorphism

The cytochrome P-450 enzyme system plays a major role in the oxidative metabolism of most drugs. With the recent advances in molecular cloning techniques about 20 human forms of cytochrome P-450 have been identified, each with distinct although overlapping substrate specificities (Gonzalez, 1992). Of these the cytochromes CYP1A2, CYP2A5, CYP2B6, CYP2C, CYP2D6, CYP2E1 and CYP3A have all been shown to metabolise clinically important drugs (Cholerton *et al.*, 1992). This is schematically shown in Figure 2.1 with the circles representing the different enzymes.

Of these enzymes CYP2D6 metabolises debrisoquine and sparteine, as well as numerous other compounds. From Figure 2.1 it may be deduced that individuals who lack CYP2D6 activity (PM's) may exhibit quite normal metabolism towards other substrates which are primarily oxidised by other cytochrome P-450 enzymes.

The human CYP2D gene cluster is localised on the long arm of chromosome 22 and DNA sequencing studies on genomic DNA from poor metabolisers of debrisoquine allows the identification of three

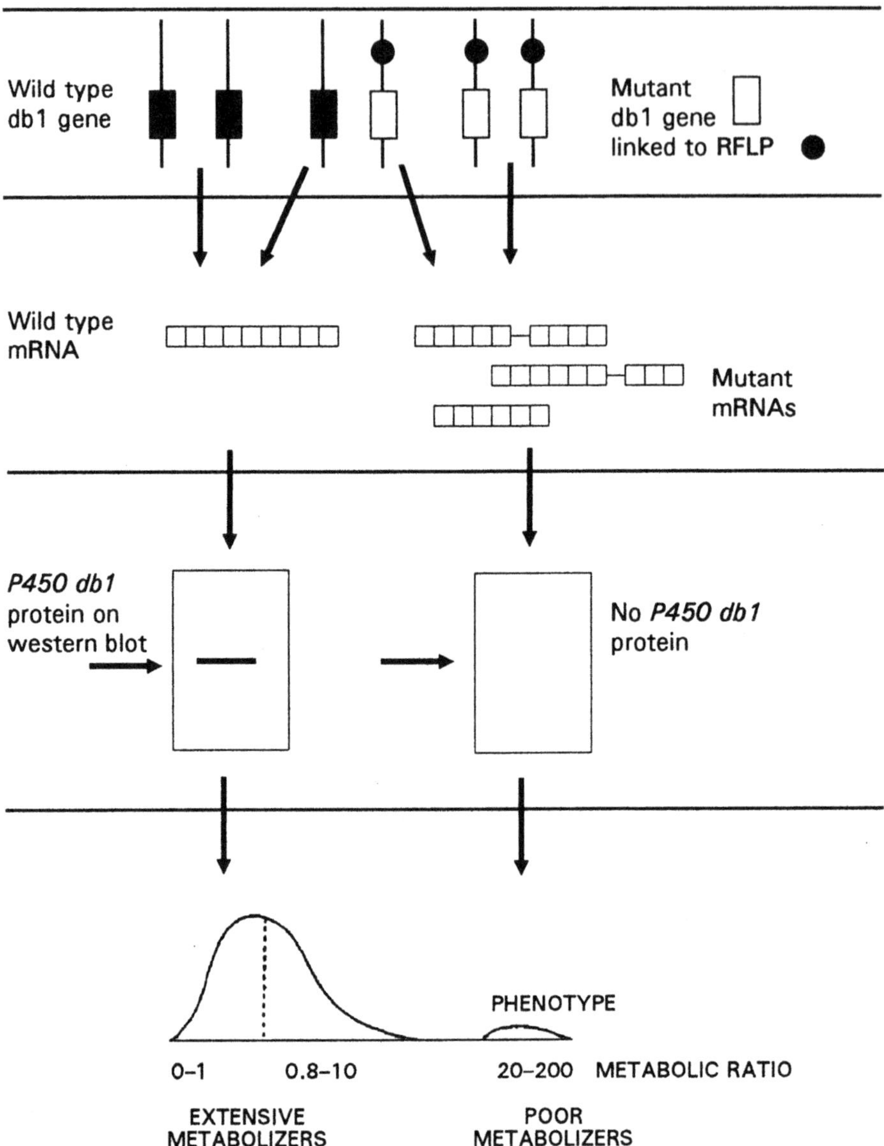

Figure 2.2 Molecular characterisation of the debrisoquine/sparteine polymorphism. The scheme gives an idea how different splicing defects may cause mutant mRN which yield no detectable P-450IID6 (P-450db1) protein and result in the debrisoquine poor metaboliser phenotype. Mutated alleles of the P-450IID6 (P-450db1) gene can be detected in genomic DNA of poor metabolisers. Reproduced from Meyer *et al.* (1992) with permission.

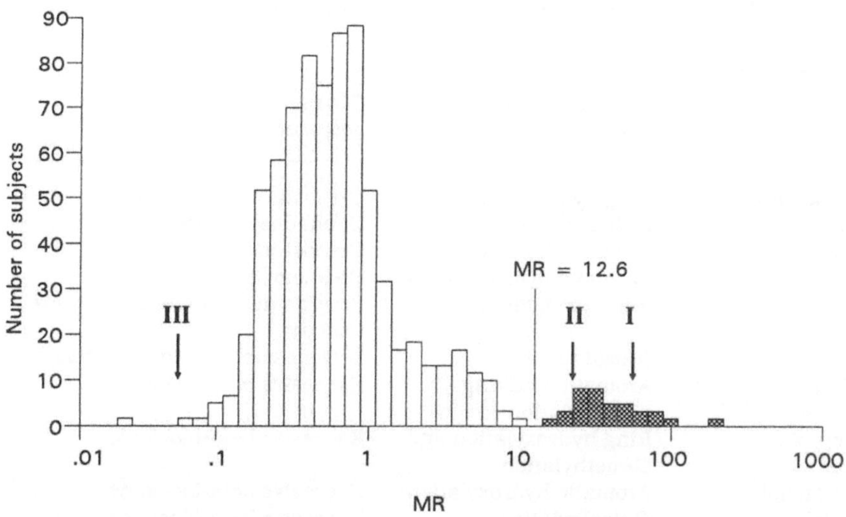

Figure 2.3 Distribution of the metabolic ratios (MR) between the urinary excretions of debrisoquine and 4′-hydroxydebrisoquine in urine of 757 healthy Swedish volunteers. An antimode at MR 12.6 distinguishes rapid and slow (6%) hydroxylators. Reproduced from Steiner *et al.* (1988) with permission.

mutant alleles of the CYP2D6 locus by restriction fragment length polymorphisms (RFLP) in lymphocytic DNA (Meyer *et al.*, 1992). This led to the development of a polymerase chain reaction (PRC) based assay to "genotype" for debrisoquine/sparteine metabolism, which is now successful in the identification of approximately 95% of European poor metabolisers (Meyer *et al.*, 1992). The relationship between the genotype (mutations) and the phenotype is schematically shown in Figure 2.2 (Meyer *et al.*, 1992).

Indeed, the bimodality in the frequency distribution of the metabolic ratio of debrisoquine (or sparteine) in a population of human subjects has been observed in several studies. In Figure 2.3 an example is shown for 757 healthy Swedish subjects (Steiner *et al.*, 1988).

In this particular population the incidence of PM's was around 6%; a similar incidence (5–10%) has been observed in other Caucasian populations, but interestingly a considerably lower incidence has been observed in Chinese and Japanese population studies (0–2.3%) (Eichelbaum and Gross, 1992). Also in Egyptians, Malaysians and Saudi Arabians the incidence seems to be lower (1–3%) than among the white Caucasian populations.

Table 2.1 Drugs with their metabolic reactions affected by the debriso-quine/sparteine polymorphism

Drug	Metabolic reaction affected	Clinical effect in poor metabolisers
Debrisoquine	Ring hydroxylation	Orthostatic hypotension
Encainide	O-demethylation	Usual dose ineffective
Guanoxan	Aromatic hydroxylation	Orthostatic hypotension
Indoramine	Aromatic hydroxylation	CNS toxicity
Perhexiline	Aliphatic hydroxylation	Peripheral neuropathy, hepato-toxicity
Sparteine	N-oxidation	Uterine contraction, CNS toxicity
Bufuralol	Aromatic and ring hydroxylation	Excessive beta-blockade
Metoprolol	Ring hydroxylation and O-methylation	Excessive beta-blockade
Propranolol	Aromatic hydroxylation	Excessive beta-blockade
Timolol	O-dealkylation	Excessive beta-blockade
Amitriptyline	N-demethylation	Possible CNS toxicity
Desipramine	Aromatic hydroxylation	Possible CNS toxicity
Dextromethorphan	O-demethylation	Possible CNS toxicity
Imipramine	Aromatic hydroxylation	Possible CNS toxicity
Nortriptyline	Ring hydroxylation	Possible CNS toxicity
Phenacetin	O-demethylation	Methaemoglobinaemia
Phenformin	Aromatic hydroxylation	Lactic acidosis

Adapted from La Du (1992).

Phenotyping in European countries generally occurs by giving a test dose of either debrisoquine or sparteine. In several other countries, however, these compounds are not available and the antitussive agent dextromethorphan represents a suitable alternative (Dayer, 1990).

Clinical implications

CYP2D6 is able to metabolise numerous substrates other than the probe drugs debrisoquine, sparteine and dextromethophan. A wide variety of different C-oxidations (aromatic, alicyclic, aliphatic) as well as O-dealkylations are catalysed by this enzyme. A common feature of these compounds is the presence of a basic nitrogen atom, but prediction of which drug will or will not be subject to polymorphic oxidation on the basis of structural considerations alone is currently not possible. Progress, however, is made in this direction by using molecular modelling techniques (Koymans *et al.*, 1992).

In Table 2.1 a (non-exhaustive) list is presented of several drugs whose metabolism is (partially) affected by the debrisoquine/sparteine (DB/SP) polymorphism, i.e. of which a specific metabolic pathway co-segregates with that of DB/SP oxidation. In addition, it has been indicated in this Table which unusual clinical effects have been observed in particular in subjects that had been phenotyped as PM's for DB/SP (La Du, 1992).

As already indicated, this list is far from complete but it is a good illustration of the potential clinical implications in the PM's if they are being treated with the same doses as the extensive metabolisers (EM's). Whether or not a deficient pathway in the metabolism of certain drugs has clinical relevance obviously depends on the relative importance of the affected pathway to the overall elimination of the compound (differences in the pharmacokinetics of parent compound between EM's and PM's) and the therapeutic window of the drug, i.e. the relationship between drug concentrations and desirable versus adverse effects. Theoretically the following therapeutic implications may be anticipated (Eichelbaum and Gross, 1992; Wilkinson, 1989):

A. *In PM's*: Reduced first-pass metabolism leading to considerably increased bioavailability (higher C_{max} and AUC) that is associated with exaggerated drug response; examples: debrisoquine and some β-blocking agents.

B. *In PM's*: Reduced rate of drug elimination leading to prolonged elimination half-life, drug accumulation during chronic dosing and increased pharmacological response and drug toxicity; examples: perhexeline and some tricyclic antidepressants.

C. *In PM's*: Prodrug is not activated, i.e. active metabolite is not formed leading to lack of or reduced therapeutic efficacy; examples: encainide with active metabolite 3-methoxy-*O*-desmethylencainide and codeine with active metabolite morphine.

D. *In EM's*: Drug interactions with other compounds which are metabolised by or are substrate of CYP2D6; examples: quinidine and propafenone. By using quinidine one may even inhibit the rate of metabolism of the probe drugs DB and SP in EM's to an extent that they switch to the apparent PM status.

The importance of the DB/SP polymorphism in the clinical application of tricyclic antidepressants and of some neuroleptics has recently been discussed separately by Sjöqvist (1992), whereas Lennard (1992) did this for β-blocking agents.

For obvious reasons compromised drug safety in PM's is a major concern in considering the clinical relevance of DB/SP polymorphism and examples have been given that this is rightly so for some drugs. It is still important, however, to also recognise that considerable inter-individual variability in drug metabolising activity exists within both phenotypic groups and in particular among the EM's (see Figure 2.3). Very rapid hydroxylators of debrisoquine have been described (metabolic ratio <0.1; see for example subject III in Figure 2.3), which require far higher than usual doses of tricyclic antidepressant agents to achieve a therapeutic effect (Bertilsson *et al.*, 1985; Ibid 1993). Clinically it should be regarded as equally relevant to detect and distinguish between patients at the extreme ends of unimodal distribution as between patients belonging to the different modes of a bimodal distribution. It is the magnitude rather than the origin of the variability that determines the clinical relevance and therefore there is no fundamental contrast between genetic factors (polymorphism) and environmental factors causing variability in the rate of drug metabolism (Breimer, 1989). This observation of course extends to any metabolic reaction other than oxidation.

Consequences in ADME studies during drug development

In 1989 a European conference was held on "Pharmacogenetics" under the auspices of COST which stands for European Cooperation in the field of Scientific and Technical Research. The meeting was organised by the management committee of the COST-B1 project, entitled "Criteria for the choice and definition of healthy volunteers and patients for Phase I and Phase II studies in drug development". This committee had been discussing the issue of polymorphism in oxidative drug metabolism on a regular basis since 1985. At this meeting the state of the art was discussed with respect to the molecular and enzymatic basis, *in vivo* phenotyping, clinical relevance and consequences for drug development and drug regulation. The latter topics were discussed by representatives of European pharmaceutical industries and regulatory authorities. The proceedings of the conference were published by the EC – Directorate General Science, Research and Development in 1990 (Alvan *et al.*, 1990) and contain both the review lectures, as well as the discussions among the participants. The overall consensus with respect to the consequences of polymorphism in drug oxidation in drug development (ADME studies) was that it should be considered and taken into account as early as possible in the preclinical phases.

The existence of genetic polymorphism should be considered as a special case of inter-subject variability and should not be a reason *per se* for not further developing or marketing a drug, unless drug safety and/or efficacy would be highly compromised. After all, many clinically important drugs are on the market which exhibit this type of polymorphism in their metabolism, although this was recognised in retrospect only. Similar views have been expressed in a paper by Balant *et al.*, (1989).

Major advances have already been made in the development of *in vitro methodology* using *human* microsomes, hepatocytes, cell lines, purified enzymes and specific antibodies that allow the detection of potential metabolic pathways that are primarily catalysed by human CYP2D6 or other specific enzymes. This should occur during early preclinical drug development, in parallel to the usual ADME studies in laboratory animals and the identification process of major metabolites (metabolic screen). CYP2D6 and other P-450 enzymes have been expressed in cell lines and have been purified and this offers the tools to study the metabolism of new drugs by specific enzymes and to identify the particular pathways that are catalysed. Furthermore, studies in human liver microsomes (preferably of known phenotype or genotype) may elucidate different parallel pathways in the metabolism of a compound and the use of antibodies against CYP2D6 will allow a polymorphic pathway to be identified. This approach may also indicate whether or not this pathway is quantitatively a major one in the overall metabolism of the compound, although this definitely requires confirmation *in vivo*. Alternatively, *in vitro* inhibition studies with known substrates (or high binding affinity) of specific enzymes have proved to be very helpful in assessing the relative contribution of a particular pathway to the total metabolism of a compound. For CYP2D6, for example, quinidine may be used and specific inhibitors of other enzymes have been indicated in Figure 2.1. The identification of a specific enzyme catalysing an important metabolic pathway of a new drug may also be very helpful in predicting which drug–drug interactions are likely to occur and thereby help to plan the appropriate studies *in vivo*. The *in vitro* strategy as discussed allows for an early recognition of the fact that a new drug will be subject to genetic polymorphism in part of its metabolism. If the drug is judged to be of great therapeutic potential this should not necessarily lead to stopping further development. Alternatively a "back-up" compound not exhibiting polymorphism may be preferred for further investigation.

The information on a new compound obtained preclinically should be used to optimise Phase I and Phase II clinical studies. If the preclinical data strongly suggest that the metabolism of the drug is subject to the DB/SP (or mephenytoin) genetic polymorphism, the early investigations in man should be conducted in subjects of both EM and PM phenotype (phenotyped panel approach). This allows the assessment of the degree of genetic variability in drug metabolism and pharmacokinetics in relation to phenotype. A major difference between EM's and PM's is only expected if clearance is dependent on the rate of one major oxidative route only. Phenotyping is possible either by giving a single probe drug detecting a specific polymorphism, or by combining, for example, sparteine, mephenytoin and other probe drugs to obtain a more complete picture of the metabolic status of an individual subject ("cocktail" approach) (Breimer and Schellens, 1990). In Phase I also the first information on drug response may be obtained in relationship to dose and/or concentration and a first indication may be obtained on the steepness of dose or concentration effect relationship and thereby on the pharmacological relevance of the polymorphism. This will be further substantiated in phenotyped patients in Phase II trials. Subsequently, it has to be decided whether or not phenotyping and dose adjustments are indicated in Phase III studies in relatively large patient populations.

References

Alván G, Balant LP, Bechtel, PR, Boobis AR, Gram LF and Pithan K (eds) (1990). *Proceedings European Consensus Conference on Pharmacogenetics*. Commission of the European Communities (Co-ordinated Action COST B1), Luxembourg.

Andersson T, Regardh CG, Lou YC, Zhang Y, Dahl ML and Bertilsson L (1992). Polymorphic hydroxylation of S-mephenytoin and omeprazole metabolism in Caucasian and Chinese subjects. *Pharmacogenetics*, **2**:25–31.

Balant LP, Gundert-Remy U, Boobis AR and von Bahr Ch (1989). Relevance of genetic polymorphism in drug metabolism in the development of new drugs. *Eur J Clin Pharmacol*, **36**: 551–554.

Bertilsson L, Aberg-Wistedt A, Gustafsson LL, Nordin C (1985). Extremely rapid hydroxylation of debrisoquine: a case report with implications for treatment with nortriptyline and other tricyclic antidepressants. *Ther Drug Monit*, **7**:478–480.

Bertilsson L, Henthorn TK, Sanz E, Tybring G, Säwe J and Villén T (1989). Importance of genetic factors in the regulation of diazepam metabolism: relationship to S-mephenytoin, but not debrisoquine, hydroxylation phenotype. *Clin Pharmacol Ther*, **45**:348–355.

Bertilsson L, Dahl M-L, Sjöqvist F, Asberg-Wistedt A, Humble M, Johansson I, Lundquist E and Ingelman-Sundberg M (1993). Molecular basis for rational megaprescribing in ultrarapid hydroxylators of debrisoquine. *Lancet*, **341**:63.

Breimer, DD (1983). Interindividual variations in drug disposition. Clinical implications and methods of investigation. *Clin Pharmacokin*, **8**:371–377.

Breimer DD (1990). Potential clinical relevance of the interplay between genetic and environmental factors. In: Alván *et al.* (eds) pp. 69–80.

Breimer DD and Schellens JHM (1990). A "cocktail" strategy to assess *in vivo* oxidative drug metabolism in humans. *Trends Pharmacol Sci*, **11**:223–225.

Cholerton S, Daly AK and Idle JR (1992). The role of individual human cytochromes P-450 in drug metabolism and clinical response. *Trends Pharmacol Sci*, **13**:434–439.

Dayer P (1990). Advantages and drawbacks of probe drugs for the assessment of the phenotypic expression of cytochrome P-450 DB1 (P450IID6). In: Alván *et al.* (eds), pp. 33–42.

Eichelbaum M and Gross AS (1992). The genetic polymorphism of debrisoquine/sparteine metabolism – clinical aspects. In: Kalow W (ed.), pp. 625–648

Eichelbaum M, Spannbrucker N, Steincke B and Dengler HJ (1979). Defective *N*-oxidation of sparteine in man: a new pharmacogenetic defect. *Eur J Clin Pharmacol*, **16**:153.

Gonzalez FJ (1992). Human cytochromes P450: problems and prospects. *Trends Pharmacol Sci*, **13**:346–352.

Kalow W (ed.) (1992). *Pharmacogenetics of Drug Metabolism*. Pergamon Press, New York.

Koymans LMH, Vermeulen NPE, van Acker SABE, te Koppele JM, Heykants JJP, Lavrijsen K, Meuldermans W and Donné-Op den Kelder GM (1992). A predictive model for substrates of cytochrome P-450 debrisoquine (2D6). *Chem Res Toxicol*, **5**:211–219.

Küpfer A and Preisig P (1984). Pharmacogenetics of mephenytoin: a new hydroxylation polymorphism in man. *Eur J Clin Pharmacol*, **26**:753–759.

La Du BN (1992). Overview of pharmacogenetics. In: Kalow W (ed.), pp. 1–12.

Lennard MS (1992). The polymorphic oxidation of beta-adrenoreceptor antagonists. In: Kalow W (ed.), pp. 701–720.

Mahgoub A, Idle JR, Dring LG, Lancester R and Smith RL (1977). Polymorphic hydroxylation of debrisoquine in man. *Lancet*, **2**:584–586.

Meyer UA, Skoda RC, Zanger UM, Heim M and Broly F (1992). The genetic polymorphism of debrisoquine/sparteine metabolism – molecular mechanisms. In: Kalow W (ed.), pp. 609–623.

Price Evans DA (1992). *N*-Acetyltransferase. In: Kalow W (ed.), pp. 95–178.

Sjöqvist F (1992). Pharmacogenetic factors in the metabolism of tricyclic antidepressants and some neuroleptics. In: Kalow W (ed.), p. 689–700.

Steiner E, Bertilsson L, Säwe J, Bertling I and Sjöqvist F (1988). Polymorphic debrisoquine hydroxylation in 757 Swedish subjects. *Clin Pharmacol Ther,* **44**:431–435.

Tucker GT, Silas JH, Iyun AO, Lennard MS and Smith AJ (1977). Polymorpic hydroxylation of debrisoquine. *Lancet,* **2**:718.

Vasko MR, Bell RD, Daly DD and Pippenger CE (1980). Inheritance of phenytoin hypometabolism: a kinetic study of one family. *Clin Pharmacol Ther,* **27**:96–103.

Wilkinson GR (1989).Pharmacogenetic factors responsible for variability in drug disposition. In: Breimer DD, Crommelin JJ and Midha KK, (eds) *Topics in Pharmaceutical Sciences*, Fédération Internationale Pharmaceutique, The Hague, pp. 541–554.

Wilkinson GR, Guengerich FP and Branch RA (1992). Genetic polymorphism of S-mephenytoin hydroxylation. In: Kalow W (ed.), p. 657–685

3
Inter-ethnic differences in dose–response studies

LUC P BALANT and PIERRE BECHTEL

Summary

1. Currently, it is unclear how frequent or widespread genetic differences are with respect to drug metabolism nor is it always apparent how these differences are influenced by culture, life-style or choice of foods. Therefore, questions are raised as to what are the medical and toxicological consequences of these ethnic differences.

2. Inter-ethnic investigations in Phase I and II studies should provide information on dose–concentration–response relationships. The overall benefit of these investigations of pharmacokinetics and pharmacodynamics in both preclinical and clinical studies can produce an early identification of optimal dosing regimens thus shortening the overall time for drug development.

3. If *in vitro* data obtained with human microsomes or human hepatocytes indicate that the metabolism of a new compound might be under the control of a known genetic polymorphism, it is now well accepted that the first studies in healthy volunteers should ideally be performed in a panel consisting both of extensive and poor metabolisers. If the difference between the two groups shows potential clinical significance, special care must be taken in the development of the new compound. If the contrary is true, drug development may generally proceed without this requirement.

4. However, if a drug product is developed involving essentially healthy subjects and patients of a single racial group and if the product is to be commercialised in a geographic area where another racial group is predominant, some precautions must be taken as far as safety and efficacy are concerned.

Introduction

Kalow (1992) has stated, "*...that there are inter-ethnic differences in drug-metabolising capacity is now a well established fact... Nevertheless, it is not clear how frequent or how widespread genetic differences are, nor is it clear how many differences are dependent on culture, lifestyle, or choice of foods...*". Accordingly, questions are raised as "*to what extent these differences are of medical and toxicological consequences?... Whether, or under what circumstances, some of the recognised, genetically controlled differences in metabolic capacity can be ignored, and when they need to be considered in order to protect important segments of a population from harmful effects of drugs...?*". However, differences in drug response are also of crucial importance, and they will be addressed in order to explore how the known inter-ethnic differences in drug response can be used to propose *ad hoc* strategies for the study of dose–response relationships.

In the context of worldwide drug development the potential existence of inter-ethnic differences in behaviour and action of drugs which have not yet been discovered is probably as important as for those which are already discovered. However, the literature on this subject is naturally limited and one must rely for the most part on anecdotal reports. It is thus not surprising to find that it is usual to guess rather than to plan which action should be undertaken in order to provide drugs with maximum efficiency and minimum side-effects in various continents and regions.

Basic definitions

Pharmacoanthropology

Kalow (1984) has proposed that pharmacoanthropology be defined as the branch of pharmacology or clinical pharmacology that deals with inter-ethnic differences in *response to* or *metabolism of* drugs. The reference to anthropology is meant to indicate that the inquiry is of scientific rather than political nature, and is not biased by considering only genetic or only cultural factors. It thereby differs from pharmacogenetics which deals specifically with hereditary variations in drug metabolism.

In classical genetics three main human races are recognised: the Caucasians, the Negroids and the Mongoloids. In addition, two other races comprising less individuals are distinguished: the Bushmen and the Australian aborigines. However, as far as drug development in concerned, each of the large races consists of subgroups (e.g.

characterised by well defined genetic polymorphisms in drug metabolism) and any group tested will be somewhat different from the "average" Caucasian, "average" Mongoloid, or "average" Negroid (Kalow, 1992). The question then arises to what extent should races be considered when testing new drugs in the context of a worldwide development. Since it is not possible to test drugs under all possible situations, *ad hoc* strategies must be developed.

In order to concentrate on issues related to drug development, licensing and registration, this paper will dwell more on conceptual issues than on the scientific basis of inter-ethnic differences in drug metabolism and response. Most of the statements will thus represent personal opinions of the authors rather than established regulatory guidelines, which are essentially non-existent in the context of inter-ethnic differences or similarities in drug behaviour and effects.

Definitions of "ethnicity" in the context of new drug development

Before discussing the pharmacokinetic and pharmacodynamic implications of "inter-ethnic" differences for new drug development, it is important to define some concepts which may have different meanings outside of the scientific field.

Species, racial or *ethnic classifications* have different significance depending on their context of use. The definitions given below are those from Churchill's Medical Dictionary (1989).

Species [Latin (from *specere* to see, observe) a sight, aspect, appearance, form, type, particular kind]. A taxonomic collection of interbreeding populations that are reproductively isolated from other such collections. A group of closely related species forms a genus.

Race [Middle French, from Italian *razza* race, kind]. A subspecies or other division or subdivision of a species. Human races are generally defined in terms of original geographic range and common hereditary traits which may be morphological, serological, haematological, immunological, or biochemical. The traditional division of mankind into several well-recognised racial types focusing on a limited range of visible characteristics tends to oversimplify and distort the picture of human variation.

Ethnic [Greek *ethnikos* (from *ethnos* a nation, people) national, of a people]. Designating the physical and cultural traits that distinguish members of one society or larger human group from members of other such groups.

Since the scope of this review is to address issues related to drug development and use in large groups of people, without regard for divisions which are merely of a tribal, linguistic or political nature, the term "racial" will be used to focus on genetic traits, whereas "ethnic" will be used to encompass also environmental factors. As an example, a difference in drug response observed in second generation Asians living in North America with the same life habits as Caucasian-Americans will be termed "racial", whereas the same observation made between Japan or China and North-America will be termed "ethnic" as long as the underlying causes (i.e. genetic and/or environmental) have not been elucidated.

Pharmacogenetics

Basically, the behaviour of all drugs is determined (at least to some extent) by genetic factors. It is thus possible to state that "pharmacogenetics" is a basic component of the inter-individual variability of all drugs. It is, however, customary to restrict the term "pharmacogenetics" when one (or more) distinct subpopulations can be identified as far as their metabolic capacities towards drugs or group of drugs are concerned. Genetic factors influencing drug metabolism can be mono- or polygenic. If they are of monogenic type, they present themselves either as polymorphisms or as rare phenotypes. A *genetic polymorphism* is a monogenic trait that exists in the population in at least two phenotypes and at least two genotypes, neither of which is rare, i.e. less frequent than 1% (Meyer *et al.*, 1990). Genetic polymorphisms of drug metabolism usually segregate the population into two groups differing in their ability to metabolise certain drugs. Individuals with a deficient metabolism are termed "poor metabolisers", as compared to "extensive metabolisers". For more information on genetic polymorphisms, consult the chapter by D.D. Breimer in the present volume.

Drugs, substances and medicinal products

Drugs may mean different entities depending on the context. The nomenclature adopted here is that of the European Community (Council Directive, 1965) according to which:

A substance is a "chemical", e.g. element, naturally occurring chemical material and chemical product obtained by structural change or synthesis. In so far as a substance shows pharmacological activity it may be termed an *"active substance"* or, if intended for use as a medicinal product, a *"drug"* or the *"active drug"*.

A medicinal product is any substance or combination of substances presented for treating or preventing disease in human beings or animals. The term drug product will be used as a synonym. It is thus conceivable, if differences in behaviour or effect are detected for a given substance in different ethnic groups, that different drug products (e.g. differences in dosing strength, rate of release etc.) must be marketed in different countries or prescribed differentially depending on the patient's ethnicity.

Phases of clinical trials during drug development

In the context of this review, *clinical trials* imply (a) systematic studies in humans designed to discover or verify the pharmacodynamics, the therapeutic effects and/or adverse reactions of medicinal products, and (b) human pharmacokinetic studies as defined by the European Communities.

Phase I trials of a new active substance in man are conducted in healthy volunteers, with a few exceptions such as cytostatic agents and immunomodulators. Phase I does not only make reference to timing in drug development, but also to a basic methodological aspect, in the sense that fate and effects of drugs are investigated in healthy volunteers. Accordingly, Phase I type studies can be performed at any time in the life cycle of a drug, for example, as bioequivalence studies after the medicinal product has been in clinical use for many years (Balant *et al.*, 1990).

Phase II trials are pilot therapeutic studies in patients. They are usually explorative (controlled or not) during Phase IIa and controlled in Phase IIb. One important objective is to provide information on dose–response relationships, or better, on dose–concentration–response relationships. The pharmacodynamic parameters thus obtained are often short-term response parameters, the so-called surrogate endpoints.

For the sake of clarity, we shall use the term *"Phase IIa"* to describe studies close in their methodology to those performed in healthy subjects, and *"Phase IIb"* those which are closer to full scale Phase III clinical trials. It is obvious that this delineation is arbitrary and that other definitions would also be adequate. This presentation will concentrate on Phase IIa investigations, whereas the companion paper (Balant *et al.*, 1994) will deal more extensively with Phase IIb clinical trials.

Phase III trials are the classical clinical trials. The implications of inter-ethnic differences in drug metabolism or action for the design and interpretation of Phase III clinical trials are discussed in the companion paper (Balant *et al.*, 1994).

Phase IV trials are performed after marketing of the final medicinal product. At this stage, clinical trials exploring new indications, new pharmaceutical formulations, new methods of administration, new dosage regimen or new target subpopulations are considered as trials of new medicinal products having similar objectives as pre-marketing trials. Such studies may consequently require trial conditions as defined for Phase I, II or III. This is particularly true for pharmacokinetic and bioavailability studies performed for product licensing from one ethnic area to another one.

Pharmacokinetics (PK) and pharmacodynamics (PD)

The concepts underlying *pharmacokinetics* in the present review are well known and suitably described in textbooks. The term "pharmacokinetics" will be used in this review as a generic term qualifying the study of the kinetics of absorption, distribution, metabolism and excretion (ADME) of substances or medicinal products active in preventing or treating human diseases.

The term pharmacodynamics is also well defined in textbooks. We shall use the combination *"concentration–effect"* to characterise studies in which a well-defined and quantifiable effect can be measured, preferably in function of concentrations of the active substance rather than administered dose. The concept *"dose–response"* will be used to characterise situations in which a given response (e.g. lowering of blood pressure under a certain value, percentage change on a depression rating scale, etc.) is analysed as a function of the prescribed or administered dose. This is clearly an arbitrary choice, but it has certain advantages in the context of inter-ethnic differences in drug action or response.

In the authors' opinion, it is clear that dose–response is the information usually needed for drug registration and prescription in daily practice. However, in order to adequately define such relationships, it is of primary importance to distinguish pharmacokinetic and pharmacodynamic sources of variability. This is best performed by the investigation of the *"dose–concentration–effect–response"* relationships. This problem has already been discussed to some extent during the First Conference on Harmonisation (Hashimoto, 1992; Naito, 1992; Wardell, 1992).

Integration of pharmacokinetic and pharmacodynamic principles in drug development

The conceptual framework

The overall benefit that the integration of pharmacokinetics (PK) and pharmacodynamics (PD) in preclinical and clinical studies can produce is an early identification of optimal dosing regimens, thus shortening the overall time of drug development (Peck *et al.* 1992). Of equal importance, the increased understanding of drug action derived from PK/PD integration leads to a more informative drug development programme, especially with regard to identification of dosage regimens that result in optimal therapeutic outcome through strategies for *individualisation of dosage*, either in individuals or in subpopulations such as patients with specific pathologies or ethnic groups.

A critical step in the complex process of drug development is to decide if animal and early human studies of drug response suggest useful clinical activity (Holford, 1992). Useful clinical activity is supported initially by demonstrating a potential therapeutic effect. A therapeutic effect may be shown by demonstrating that a significant difference exists in comparison with a placebo or a reference drug. While this kind of binary decision-making is presently the normal case in drug development, it does not describe the complexities of using a drug which are usually recognised when subsequently widely used. Accordingly, it has been advocated (Peck *et al.*, 1992) to use the pharmacokinetic/pharmacodynamic (PK/PD) approach to link dosage with knowledge of drug disposition, and coupling that with observable clinical outcomes. This paradigm is particularly useful for dose finding during Phase I and Phase II studies. Since discovery of optimal dosing regimens early in drug development may contribute to efficient drug development programmes by mitigating failed clinical trials, it is obvious that this information should be acquired early in the development process. This is even more important if registration is intended in different ethnic groups for which differences in PK and/or PD parameters may be observed.

Phase I studies

The well accepted objectives of Phase I studies are to define the initial parameters of tolerance and effect (if measurable in healthy volunteers), and their relation to dosage and relevant pharmacokinetics of the drug. These studies are also intended to optimise the drug delivery system and to probe potential drug–drug interactions that might be expected to perturb the PK/PD relationship. Accordingly, whenever possible, parallel measurements of systemic concentrations and acute effects should be performed in order to provide data for PK/PD modelling. Clearly, feedback is needed between the results obtained in patients during Phase I and Phase II bioavailability studies.

PK/PD modelling during Phase I studies is restricted to those drugs for which acute effects can be measured in healthy volunteers. Quantitative data analysis too often deals with calculation of PK parameters only and neglects simultaneous consideration of PD aspects. This is a result of the lack of appropriate pharmacological endpoints or because of the difficulty in their quantitative assessment. In addition, in many instances, such an approach is not attempted because it is felt that the measurable effects are without clinical relevance. However, in many cases it is probable that linking measured systemic drug concentrations with observations of acute toxic effects or intolerance (PD) may lead to preliminary definition of maximum safe drug concentrations and doses (Peck, 1992). Such an approach is certainly closer to the "pharmacokinetic screen" discussed in the companion paper, than to traditional PK/PD modelling using integrated models. Similar considerations apply for early Phase II clinical trials during which only a small and selected number of patients is studied.

Investigational pharmacokinetics

If *in vitro* data obtained with human microsomes or human hepatocytes indicate that the metabolism of a new compound might be under the control of a known genetic polymorphism, it is now well accepted that the first studies in healthy volunteers should ideally be performed in a panel consisting both of extensive and poor metabolisers (Balant *et al.*, 1989). If the difference between the two groups shows potential clinical significance, special care must be taken in the development of the new compound. If the contrary is true, drug development may generally proceed without this requirement. Until recently, it was customary to extend this type of targeted pharmacokinetic investigation to other ethnic groups than the main ethnic component of the country of origin of the compound. This was done only if it was evident that licensing out to countries with other ethnic majorities was a prime goal in the development of the new medication. However, with the important migrations that characterise the later part of this century it becomes increasingly evident that other strategies must be examined if the new drug product is to be marketed in multi-ethnic countries or different geographic areas.

In this context, as well as for licensing purposes, two situations may be distinguished: (a) the metabolism of the drug is under the control of a known polymorphism; and (b) no defined polymorphism has been detected. In the first case, specific study designs may be used combining ethnic groups and metaboliser status. In the second case no specific recommendations may be given at this stage of drug development and it is probably necessary to wait for Phase III studies using the pharmacokinetic screen approach (or others) in order to detect possible ethnic differences in drug metabolism and response. The following two examples serve as an illustration of the potential problems encountered if a polymorphism is detected early in drug development (bufuralol) or if a difference is found without known causes (cephoperazone).

Early in the development of bufuralol, a β-blocker, it was suspected that its metabolism was under the control of a polymorphic enzyme (Balant *et al.*, 1976). During a Phase I pharmacokinetic study, a volunteer suffered from marked orthostatic hypotension with simultaneous very high blood concentrations of parent drug, and very low concentrations of the hydroxylated metabolite. Further work by the same group confirmed this hypothesis (Dayer *et al.*, 1983, 1985). In Great Britain, investigators of the behaviour of debrisoquine, an antihypertensive drug, found that marked hypotensive response in one volunteer was due to impaired 4-hydroxylation of the drug (Mahgoub *et al.*, 1977). At about the same time, a group of physicians in Bonn observed increased side-effects associated with decreased oxidative metabolism of sparteine, an anti-arrhythmic and oxytocic drug (Eichelbaum *et al.*, 1979). Since these early observations, numerous investigations have followed, indicating that the proportion of "poor" metabolisers is about 7% in Caucasian populations (see chapter by D.D. Breimer in the present volume).

Later, the development of bufuralol was stopped because there were already a number of β-blockers available. The relatively narrow therapeutic margin combined with the sensitivity of its metabolism to the debrisoquine/sparteine type polymorphism was an additional reason for this decision.

This case is interesting since today we know the reason for the strange behaviour of the volunteer in the early pharmacokinetic experiment. It must, however, be remembered that in 1974, when this early study was performed, polymorphic metabolism was not recognised. Let us imagine that bufuralol could have been synthesised and tested in China or Japan, before being licensed out for clinical testing in USA and/or Europe. As mentioned above, among Caucasians, between 5 and 10% of subjects are classified as poor metabolisers (Alván *et al.*, 1990). This proportion drops to less than one percent in native Chinese both from Han and Mongolian origin (Lou *et al.*, 1987). Similar results were obtained with mainland Chinese from Hunan (Horai *et al.*, 1989). Three studies in native Japanese (Nakamura *et al.*, 1985; Ishizaki *et al.*, 1987; Horai *et al.*, 1989) have also shown that there is a low proportion of poor metabolisers in this population (from 0 to 2.5%). It is thus highly probable that in China or Japan, bufuralol would not have shown the adverse properties which led to the interruption of its developmental programme. This could have had important consequences in the case of its transfer to North America or Europe. It must also be remembered that bufuralol was a special case among β-blockers, having a relatively narrow therapeutic margin.

The knowledge we have today must also caution those who would be tempted to oversimplify the subject. In further studies of the debrisoquine/sparteine polymorphism, using genomic leucocyte DNA from some Chinese, and analysis of restriction fragment length polymorphisms (RFLPs), a number of Chinese with low metabolic ratios (i.e. extensive metaboliser phenotype) were shown to be genotypically poor metabolisers (Yue *et al.*, 1989). This study indicates that the antimode for a probe drug determined in one population might not be appropriate for another and that, in Chinese, the antimode for the debrisoquine metabolic ratio is probably lower than in Caucasians. The mechanism behind the dissociation between debrisoquine hydroxylation phenotype and genotype is not known. It is possible that the Chinese, in addition to debrisoquine hydroxylase (CYPIID6), have another enzyme able to hydroxylate debrisoquine. Another possibility is that the gene which is inoperative in the Caucasian poor metabolisers is operational in the Chinese, producing debrisoquine hydroxylase (Bertilsson, 1990). For more details, see the paper by D.D. Breimer in the present volume.

Whatever the relevance of pharmacogenetics, it is important to recall that it is most probable that genetic polymorphism in drug metabolism does not explain all differences in drug response found between different ethnic groups since environmental factors certainly also play an important role. In addition, it is certain (as discussed below) that pharmacodynamic differences in response exist in different groups. As an example, despite the fact that propranolol is metabolised faster in Chinese subjects than in Caucasians, the Chinese are more sensitive to the β-blocking effect. Stereoselective metabolism of the drug does not explain these differences, suggesting a pharmacodynamic cause for the increased sensitivity (Zhou and Wood, 1990).

A parenteral cephalosporin, *cefoperazone*, developed in Japan, was acquired by a US multinational pharmaceutical company for development and marketing in other countries (USA and Occidental Europe being included). The new drug had an adequate microbiological profile and an elimination half-life of more than 3 hours, permitting twice-a-day administration. This property was considered important since most drugs of the same class have a shorter half-life. In addition, elimination in Japanese healthy volunteers was about 50% by renal (CL_R = 20 ml/min) and 50% by non-renal (CL_{NR} = 20 ml/min) processes. On the first administration to Caucasian healthy volunteers (Allaz *et al.*, 1979), it was surprising to observe that the elimination half-life measured only about 1.7 hours. Pharmacokinetic analysis showed that renal clearance was identical in Japanese and Caucasian subjects, but that non-renal clearance in Caucasians was 60 ml/min, reducing renal excretion to 25% of the dose. Careful examination of the microbiological and kinetic data showed that, despite this difference, the drug was still a good candidate for twice a day administration in Caucasians, although the difference with similar drugs was not as striking as in Japanese patients. Another interesting observation was made: some hours after completing the study, 2 out of 8 volunteers showed a probable antabuse reaction when they had a "good" lunch with the money received for their participation to the study (Allaz *et al.*, 1979). This reaction, which was confirmed in later studies, had not been detected in Japan. This is probably due to the fact that 50% of the Japanese population is defective in acetaldehyde dehydrogenase and, alcohol-induced flushing being a commonly observed reaction, this interaction had not been detected during Phase I-III studies in the country of origin. On the contrary, in Switzerland where "flushes" are extremely rare, the reaction was immediately evident.

Investigational pharmacodynamics

There are some well documented cases of drugs or drug families for which inter-ethnic differences exist in terms of efficacy or tolerance. Thus, among the congenital defects, by far the most common is glucose-6-phosphate dehydrogenase deficiency. Individuals with the Mediterranean type G6PD have a more unstable enzyme than other genotypes and, therefore, a much lower overall enzyme activity than, for example, Blacks with the A-variant. Such patients are at risk of suffering from a fulminate haemolytic crisis following exposure to oxidants such as sulfa-drugs or some fava beans. Clearly the impact of this defect on the tolerance of a new drug cannot be tested in healthy volunteers and *in vitro* methods using red blood cells from sensitive subjects must be used. Such a procedure is mandatory, for example, if a new drug with a physico-chemical profile close to sulfa-drugs is to be marketed in Sardinia where the Mediterranean type of G6PD is particularly important. This is a situation in which intolerance to a drug is independent of the pharmacokinetic profile. This dramatic example emphasises, as already discussed, that pharmacodynamic aspects should not be neglected in the context of new drug development in different racial or ethnic groups, even if this aspect is usually more difficult to study than pharmacokinetic variability. One of the reasons is to be found in the fact that drugs are usually designed to correct symptoms in patients and not to elicit responses in healthy volunteers. As stated above, the situation is somewhat different for unwanted side-effects which are often observed in healthy and sick volunteers. In any case, pharmacodynamic investigations are usually better performed in Phase IIa settings.

Integration of PK/PD information

The ideal situation is when pharmacokinetic data may help to understand inter-ethnic differences in drug effects or response. However, the relationships are often more complicated than simple dose–concentration shifts. As an example, one may propose the potential difference in *stereoselective metabolism* which might occur in different ethnic groups when specific metabolism pathways are under the control of genetic polymorphisms. This may be exemplified with metoprolol, a β-blocking agent administered as a racemic mixture of its enantiomers. In preliminary reports, stereoselectivity in its disposition (Hermansson and von Bahr, 1982) was reported before it was known that metabolism is under the control of the debrisoquine/sparteine polymorphism. Later, the pharmacokinetics of its enantiomers has been investigated in panels of extensive and poor metabolisers following oral racemic administration (Lennard *et al.*, 1983). Significantly higher plasma concentrations of the active (S)(–)-enantiomer as compared to the inactive (R)(+)-enantiomer were observed in extensive metabolisers, whereas in poor metabolisers this stereoselectivity was decreased. Maximum plasma concentrations of both enantiomers were higher and the elimination half-life was longer in poor metabolisers. The results of a study in which extensive metabolisers were given an oral dose of pseudoracemic metoprolol indicate that preferential *O*-demethyl-ation of the inactive (R)(+)-enantiomer contributes to its more rapid clearance (relative to the (S)(–)-enantiomer) in this phenotypic group. This difference in metabolic rates is probably absent in poor metabolisers. Thus, not only is the overall clearance of metoprolol lower in poor metabolisers, but the ratio of the active and inactive enantiomers is also different in the two groups of subjects. This is an excellent example of pharmacokinetically important differences into drug metabolism. The main question, however, relates to the clinical relevance of this finding when one tries to deduce guidelines for the potential impact of such drug behaviour in two hypothetical ethnic groups, one comprising only extensive metabolisers and the other poor metabolisers.

As discussed by Lennard (1992), the "total plasma" metoprolol concentration β-blockade profile is shifted to the left in extensive metabolisers compared to poor metabolisers, a finding compatible with the higher plasma concentrations of the active isomer in the extensive metaboliser phenotype. Since a greater pharmacological effect would be expected in extensive metabolisers than in poor metabolisers at a given total [(R)+(S)] plasma drug concentration, the magnitude of the difference of drug effect between phenotypes would tend to be less than that indicated by the pharmacokinetics of the sum of the enantiomers. The confounding fact is that there is a large absolute difference in β-blocking action between the two phenotypes, as well as in total drug concentration. Lennard (1992) concludes that these differences cannot be explained by stereo-selectivity in the pharmacokinetics of metoprolol. At this stage of this rather complicated story, it would probably be clinically more relevant to conduct a Phase II trial in hypertensive patients from the two hypothetical ethnic groups, combined with pharmacoki-netic analysis in order to gain insight into drug behaviour in the target populations.

PK/PD integration is not possible

It must also be stressed that in many cases it is not possible to derive concentration–effect or response relationships from experi-mental data in healthy volunteers. In some cases it is possible (as described in the next section) to obtain this information in patients during Phase IIa studies and in other cases only the results of Phase III clinical trials allow the confirmation of the right choice concerning the chosen dose. The next example illustrates such a situation: A substance used for the treatment of liver diseases was developed in Japan. Preclinical development was performed in different animal species and led to the conclusion that, from pharmacological and toxicological data, a dose of 600 mg per day (i.e. 10 mg/kg) was adequate for clinical trials in Japan. Systemic concentrations were not available for comparison between animal species and humans (Luc P. Balant, personal observation). When the drug was acquired by a European multinational company, one of the first steps was to compare the ADME profile between Japanese and Caucasian healthy volunteers. The behaviour was indeed identical in the two groups (Luc P. Balant, personal observation). However, in Caucasians weighing generally closer to 75 kg than to 60 kg, the question was raised as to the dosage regimen. Since the elimination half-life was relatively short, one could think that steady-state concentrations (i.e. systemic clearance) was not the most important factor for drug response at the hepatic level and, accordingly, a dose of 750 mg/day was chosen for clinical trials in Europe in order to be consistent with the Japanese hypothesis. As a consequence, the Japanese formulation could not be used and a formulation had to be developed in Europe, tested for stability, and a bioequivalence trial performed before clinical trials could be started. The consequence was an important delay (as foreseen when the decision for 750 mg was taken) in the development programme. This case is interesting in the sense that it was not a difference in metabolic clearance which was a cause of concern, but body weight.

Environmental factors

As stated previously, inter-ethnic investigations should provide information on dose–concentration–response relationships. In this context, it is particularly important to obtain kinetic information in order to distinguish between *pharmacodynamic* and *pharmacokinetic* factors. However, as illustrated by a study with angiotensin I in healthy Black and White volunteers (Joubert and Brandt, 1990), *environmental factors* should also be considered. The study was conducted in South Africa in order to explore the well documented fact that Black hypertensives tend to respond poorly to some antihypertensive medications. In this study, Blacks exhibited a significantly greater angiotensin I sensitivity than Whites. Plasma renin activities were similar in the two groups and could thus not explain the observed differences. On the other hand, Blacks had significantly higher urinary sodium values and it was thus concluded that the differences in the two groups could be due largely to differences in dietary sodium intake. This study elegantly underlines the necessity to record all information potentially useful for data interpretation. It also indirectly shows that pharmacokinetic data must be obtained. As a matter of fact, had no sodium-effect been detected, the absence of data on plasma concentrations of the angiotensin I would have made data interpretation very difficult. In the present case, kinetics of the active substance was apparently not involved; this is, however, not always the case, as previously discussed.

Phase IIa studies

Clearly, as stated in the definitions, surrogate endpoints are often used in order to define dose–concentration–effect relationships. This may be the case for antihypertensive medicines for which noradrenaline-stimulation tests may be performed. Such investigations are certainly of great interest for the investigation of new drugs. However, in many cases clinical measurements closer to the real endpoint are preferable. This is the case for blood pressure measurements in antihypertensive medications, even if the ultimate criterion is survival.

Investigational pharmacokinetics

Usually purely pharmacokinetic problems can adequately be solved in healthy volunteers with the exception of a few drugs such as cytostatics or high potency neuroleptics. Haloperidol is a good example of the fact that only pharmacokinetic studies in patients could demonstrate significant kinetic differences in different ethnic groups. As an example, in a study performed in North America, haloperidol plasma concentrations among Chinese, Caucasian, and African-American groups did not significantly differ in order to achieve similar clinical response. However, the haloperidol dosage required for the Caucasian and African-American groups were significantly greater than what was needed for the Chinese group to achieve comparable plasma levels (Jann *et al.*, 1993).

Dose–response relationships

Antihypertensive medications are good examples of drugs for which dose–response studies can be performed and one point of great therapeutic interest is the detection for White and Black patients of the class of drug which will show efficacy in a maximum number of patients. Such a study has, for example, been performed by Materson *et al.* (1993) in North America in African- and Caucasian-Americans. They compared placebo, hydrochlorothiazide, atenolol, captopril, clonidine, diltiazem and prazosin and found the expected differences in response rates for the two racial groups. However, age had also a prominent effect in determining efficacy as exemplified by the comparison of "younger" and "older" Whites and Blacks.

PK/PD integration

In some situations, kinetics and dynamics are closely related and it is then relatively easy to detect the reasons of inter-ethnic differences in drug action. As an example, response to hydralazine therapy is dependent upon the acetylation phenotype. The hypotensive effect of hydralazine is greater in patients who acetylate the drug slowly and the lupus erythematosus-like syndrome produced by hydralazine occurs almost exclusively in those with slow acetylation.

In other cases the relationship between pharmacokinetics and pharmacodynamics is less obvious as demonstrated for the so-called mephenytoin polymorphism. Studies in Chinese and Japanese (Nakamura *et al.*, 1985; Horai *et al.*, 1989) have shown that 15% to 22% of these individuals are poor metabolisers of *S*-mephenytoin, whereas the proportion is less than 5% among Caucasians (Küpfer and Preisig, 1984). Although this polymorphism has been found to be of little clinical relevance for some time, the situation might change. For example, the finding that the metabolism of diazepam (mainly *N*-demethylation) and desmethyl-diazepam (mainly *C*-hydroxylation to oxazepam) is related to *S*-mephenytoin hydroxylation, but not to debrisoquine hydroxylation (Bertilsson *et al.*, 1989), together with the fact that there are more poor metabolisers of *S*-mephenytoin in Orientals than in Caucasians could be of great interest (Sanz *et al.*, 1989). Ghoneim and co-authors (1981) had indeed shown that Orientals had a lower metabolic clearance than Caucasians. Interestingly, in another study it was noted that "many Hong-Kong physicians routinely prescribe smaller diazepam doses for Chinese than for white Caucasians" (Kumana *et al.*, 1987). In the case of diazepam, the therapeutic margin is wide. Accordingly, even if a genetic polymorphism in drug metabolism should be confirmed as a major determinant in inter-individual variability for a new drug similar to diazepam, its clinical relevance would be relatively difficult to assess and it might thus well escape detection, even during drug development in different ethnic groups.

Dose-finding studies in the context of product licensing

If a drug product is developed involving essentially healthy subjects and patients of a single racial group, and if the product is to be commercialised in a geographic area where another racial group is predominant, some precautions must be taken as far as safety and efficacy are concerned. The same measures should be taken if a drug product is licensed from a parent company to its subsidiary or if the agreement is reached between two independent corporations. As an example, Darmansjah and Muchtar (1992) have listed a number of drugs which display a specific action pattern in Indonesia as compared to Europe or North America: a formulation of lesser strength had to be introduced for prochlorperazine used as an antiemetic; lower doses of chlorpromazine are used for the treatment of schizophrenia and similar measures had to be taken with sympathomimetic and β-adrenergic blocking drugs. The same authors also reported pharmacokinetic differences for rifampicin and diazepam and concluded that *"Clinicians and those who conduct trials in Asia should be aware of these differences in drug response, and the industry should be encouraged to look at the problem more thoroughly"*.

In 1979, Katz, discussing methodological problems involved in the "transcultural" development and use of psychotropic medications and, focusing on East (i.e. Asia) versus West (i.e. Europe and North America) differences, asked the following questions: *"Can a drug which is found to be effective in one country be used equally well but in a significantly smaller dosage in another country? Must clinicians be sensitive to expected differences when applying the result of a clinical trial in one country to other national settings, particularly when the other settings are culturally quite different?"* Katz then concluded that *"Despite increasing concern over the past 20 years with these practical problems, there has been little scientific action directed toward solving them"*. The impetus given to pharmacogenetics and inter-ethnic studies by the discovery of the debrisoquine/sparteine and mephenytoin polymorphisms seems to have changed this attitude.

In this context it is appropriate to mention the European Co-ordinated Action COST B1 which resulted in 1989 in the European Consensus Conference on Pharmacogenetics which was attended by scientists from academia, the pharmaceutical industry and regulatory agencies. The conference aimed at reaching a consensus on optimal approaches to deal with polymorphic drug metabolism, particularly with regard to drug development and dealt also with the problem of inter-ethnic differences in drug metabolism and response (Bertilsson, 1990).

Studies in healthy volunteers

It may be advantageous to perform, at an early stage, comparative pharmacokinetic trials in the target populations. There are no specific guidelines for such studies. It is, however, probably wise to use the same pharmaceutical formulation as administered in key pharmacokinetic trials in the country of origin. The protocol should be as close as possible to some reference protocol used to determine the pharmacokinetic "Fingerprint" (Balant *et al.*, 1990) and measurable pharmacodynamic effects in the population of origin. Blood concentration curves, urinary excretion and metabolic patterns should be determined under identical conditions.

It could be argued that it would be preferable to conduct the study in parallel in one single setting in order to minimise variables. As an example, one could study Caucasian Americans and Americans of Japanese origin in the United States. Such a study design has the advantage of homogeneity, but it does not take into account non-genetic factors such as food or environmental effects. The alternative is to compare two groups of subjects studied simultaneously in two locations or to use a "historical" control cohort.

Studies in patients

The same considerations as those expressed above in the context of worldwide development apply in the context of licensing a drug product from one ethnic setting to another. One may once again emphasise the importance of some form of pharmacokinetic information being obtained in such studies. Such data are important not only in order to understand possible inter-ethnic differences, but also to provide a rational basis for potential dosage regimen modification or dosage strength changes.

Conclusions

Pharmacogenetic differences in drug behaviour and effects can be studied in two totally different situations: (a) the drug is under the control of a known polymorphism or pharmacodynamic differences are well documented; and (b) nothing is known about polymorphism regulating enzymes or receptors. In both cases, it must be recognised that differences in the proportion of subjects of one or another phenotype in different racial groups will induce differences in drug response. Interethnicity provides the additional dimension of environmental or life style factors. A number of combinations of these factors is possible and it is not possible to give guidelines that would be valid in all occasions.

References

Allaz AF, Dayer P, Fabre J, Rudhardt M, Balant L (1979). Pharmacocinétique d'une nouvelle céphalosporine, la céfopérazone. *Schweiz Med Wochenschr*, **109**:1999–2005.

Alván G, Bechtel P, Iselius L and Gundert-Remy U (1990). Hydroxylation polymorphisms of debrisoquine and mephenytoin in European populations. *Eur J Clin Pharmacol*, **39**:533–537.

Balant L, Gorgia A, Tschopp JM, Revillard C and Fabre J (1976). Pharmacocinétique de deux médicaments bêta-bloquants: Détection d'une anomalie pharmacogénétique? *Schweiz Med Wochenschr*, **106**:1403–1407.

Balant LP, Gundert-Remy U, Boobis AR and von Bahr Ch (1989). Relevance of genetic polymorphism in drug metabolism in the development of new drugs. *Eur J Clin Pharmacol*, **36**:551–554.

Balant LP, Roseboom H and Gundert-Remy U (1990). Pharmacokinetic criteria for drug research and development. In: Testa B (ed.) *Advances in Drug Research*. Academic Press, London, pp. 1–139.

Balant LP, Gex-Fabry M and Balant-Gorgia A (1994). Implications for the design and interpretation of Phase III clinical trials. In: Walker SR, Lumley CE and McAuslane JAN (eds) *The Relevance of Ethnic Factors in the Clinical Evaluation of Medicines*. Kluwer Academic Publishers, Lancaster, pp. 199–216.

Bertilsson L, Henthorn TK, Sanz E, Tybring G, Säwe J and Villén T (1989). Importance of genetic factors in the regulation of diazepam metabolism: Relationship to S-mephenytoin, but not debrisoquine, hydroxylation phenotype. *Clin Pharmacol Ther*, **45**:348–355.

Bertilsson L (1990). Interethnic differences in drug oxidation polymorphism. In: Alván G, Balant LP, Bechtel PR, Boobis AR, Gram LF and Pithan

F (eds) *European Consensus on Pharmacogenetics*. Commission of the European Communities (Coordinated Action COST B1), Luxembourg, pp. 171–178.

Breimer DD (1994). Genetic polymorphisms in drug metabolism: clinical implications and consequences in ADME studies. In: Walker SR, Lumley CE and McAuslane JAN (eds) *The Relevance of Ethnic Factors in the Clinical Evaluation of Medicines*. Kluwer Academic Publishers, Lancaster, pp. 13–26.

Darmansjah I, Muchtar A (1992). Dose–response variation among different populations. *Clin Pharmacol Ther*, **52**:449–452.

Dayer P, Balant L, Courvoisier F, Küpfer A, Kubli A, Gorgia A and Fabre J (1982). The genetic control of bufuralol metabolism in man. *Eur J Drug Metab Pharmacokin*, **7**:73–77.

Dayer P, Balant L, Küpfer A, Courvoisier F and Fabre J (1983). Contribution of the genetic status of oxidative metabolism to variability in the plasma concentrations of beta-adrenoceptor blocking agents. *Eur J Clin Pharmacol*, **24**:797–799.

Dayer P, Balant, Küpfer A, Striberni R and Leemann T (1985). Effect of oxidative polymorphism (debrisoquine/sparteine type) on hepatic first-pass metabolism of bufuralol. *Eur J Clin Pharmacol*, **28**:317–320.

Eichelbaum M, Spannbrucker N, Steincke B and Dengler HJ (1979). Defective *N*-oxidation of sparteine in man: A new pharmacogenetic defect. *Eur J Clin Pharmacol*, **16**:183–187.

Evans DAP (1992). *N*-Acetyltransferase. In: Kalow W (ed.) *Pharmacogenetics of Drug Metabolism*. Pergamon Press, New York, pp. 95–178.

Ghoneim MM, Korttila K, Chiang CK, Jacobs L, Schoenwald RD, Mewaldt SP and Kabaya KO (1981). Diazepam effects and kinetics in Caucasians and Orientals. *Clin Pharmacol Ther*, **29**:749–756.

Hashimoto S (1992). Dose finding: Key issues. In: d'Arcy PF and Harron DWG (eds) *Proceedings of The First International Conference on Harmonisation, Brussels, 1991*. The Queen's University of Belfast, pp. 491–495.

Hermansson J and von Bahr Ch (1982). Determination of (R)- and (S)-alprenolol and (R)- and (S)-metoprolol diastereoisomeric derivatives in human plasma by reversed-phase liquid chromatography. *J Chromatogr*, **227**:113–127.

Holford NHG (1992). Parametric models for the time course of drug action: The population approach. In: Rowland M and Aarons L (eds) *New Strategies in Drug Development and Clinical Evaluation: The Population Approach*. Commission of the European Communities (Coordinated Action COST B1), Luxembourg, pp. 193–206.

Horai Y, Nakano M, Ishizaki T, Ishikawa K, Zhou HH, Zhou BJ, Lia CL and Zhang LM (1989). Metoprolol and mephenytoin oxidation polymorphisms in Far Eastern Oriental subjects: Japanese versus mainland Chinese. *Clin Pharmacol Ther*, **46**:198–207.

Ishizaki T, Eichelbaum M, Horai Y, Hashimoto K, Chiba K and Dengler HJ (1987). Evidence for polymorphic oxidation of sparteine in Japanese subjects. *Br J Clin Pharmacol*, **23**:482–485.

Jann MW, Lam YWF and Chang WH (1993). Haloperidol and reduced haloperidol plasma concentrations in different ethnic populations and interindividual variabilities in haloperidol metabolism. In: Lin KM, Poland RE and Nakasaki G (eds) *Psychopharmacology and Psychobiology of Ethnicity, Progress in Psychiatry #39*. American Psychiatric Press, Washington DC, pp. 133–152.

Joubert PH and Brandt HD (1990). Apparent racial difference in response to angiotensin I infusion. *Eur J Clin Pharmacol*, **39**:183–185.

Kalow W (1984). Pharmacoanthropology: Outline, problems, and the nature of case histories. *Fed Proc*, **43**:2314–2318.

Kalow W (1992). Pharmacoanthropology and the genetics of drug metabolism. In: Kalow W (ed.) *Pharmacogenetics of Drug Metabolism*. Pergamon Press, New York, pp. 865–877.

Katz MM *et al.* (1979). Transcultural psychopharmacology in depression: East and West. *Psychopharmacol Bull*, **15**:24–31.

Kumana CR, Lauder IJ, Chan M, Ko W and Lin HJ (1987). Differences in diazepam pharmacokinetics in Chinese and white Caucasians – Relation to body lipid stores. *Eur J Clin Pharmacol*, **32**:211–215.

Küpfer A and Preisig R (1984). Pharmacogenetics of mephenytoin: A new drug hydroxylation polymorphism in man. *Eur J Clin Pharmacol*, **26**:753–759.

Lennard MS, Tucker GT, Silas JH, Freestone S, Ramsay LE and Woods HF (1983). Differential stereoselective metabolism of metoprolol in extensive and poor debrisoquine metabolisers. *Clin Pharmacol Ther*, **34**:732–737.

Lennard MS (1992). The polymorphic oxidation of beta-adrenoceptor antagonists. In: Kalow W (ed.) *Pharmacogenetics of Drug Metabolism*. Pergamon Press, New York, pp. 701–720.

Lou YC, Ying L, Bertilsson L and Sjöqvist F (1987). Low frequency of slow debrisoquine hydroxylation in a native Chinese population. *Lancet*, **2**:852–853.

Mahgoub A, Idle JR, Dring LG, Lancester R and Smith RL (1977). Polymorphic hydroxylation of debrisoquine in man. *Lancet*, **2**, 584–586.

Materson BJ, Reda DJ, Cushman WC *et al.* (1993). Single drug therapy for hypertension in men: A comparison of six antihypertensive agents with placebo. *N Engl J Med*, 328, 914–921.

Meyer UA, Zanger UM, Grant D and Blum M (1990). Genetic polymorphisms of drug metabolism. In: Testa B (ed.) *Advances in Drug Research*. Academic Press, London, pp. 197–241.

Naito C (1992). Some problems relating to dose response trials. In: d'Arcy PF and Harron DWG (eds) *Proceedings of The First International Conference on Harmonisation, Brussels, 1991*. The Queen's University of Belfast, pp. 495–511.

Nakamura K, Goto F, Ray WA, McAllister CB, Jacqz E, Wilkinson GR and Branch RA (1985). Interethnic differences in genetic polymorphism of debrisoquin and mephenytoin hydroxylation between Japanese and Caucasian populations. *Clin Pharmacol Ther*, **38**:402–408.

Peck CC (1992). Population approach in pharmacokinetics and pharmacodynamics: FDA view. In: Rowland M and Aarons L (eds) *New Strategies in Drug Development and Clinical Evaluation: The Population Approach*. Commission of the European Communities (Coordinated Action COST B1), Luxembourg, pp. 157–168.

Peck CC *et al.* (1992). Opportunities for integration of pharmacokinetics, pharmacodynamics, and toxicokinetics in rational drug development. *Clin Pharmacol Ther*, **51**:465–473.

Sanz EJ, Villén T, Alm Ch and Bertilsson L (1989). S-mephenytoin hydroxylation phenotypes in a Swedish population determined after coadministration with debrisoquin. *Clin Pharmacol Ther*, **45**:495–499.

Wardell W (1992). What information is needed to support a dose for registration? In: d'Arcy PF and Harron DWG (eds) *Proceedings of The First International Conference on Harmonisation, Brussels, 1991*. The Queens University of Belfast, pp. 478–490.

Yue QY, Bertilsson L, Dahl-Puustinen ML, Säwe J, Sjöqvist F, Johansson I and Ingelman-Sundberg M (1989). Dissociation between debrisoquine hydroxylation phenotype and genotype among Chinese. *Lancet*, **2**:870.

Zhou HH and Wood AJJ (1990). Differences in stereoselective disposition of propranolol do not explain sensitivity differences between white and Chinese subjects: Correlation between the clearance of (–)- and (+)-propranolol. *Clin Pharmacol Ther*, **47**:719–723.

4
Evaluation methods for clinical trials of drugs in Japan which may affect ethnic differences

CHIKAYUKI NAITO

Summary

1. The frequency of adverse reactions and the usual daily dosage of drugs vary from country to country and are ascribed, in general, to ethnic differences. To date these may have been a serious hindrance to the mutual acceptance of clinical data.

2. In Japan, the clinical evaluation methodology for assessing efficacy, safety and utility have been used for some time and have been a major influence on the new drug approval process in spite of the poor scientific background to this methodology.

3. Efficacy is determined in terms of improved rating ie: marked, moderate, slight, unchanged or aggravated. Safety is assessed in terms of the degree of adverse events rated as no problem, slightly problematic, problematic and seriously problematic. Utility is evaluated by the subjective impression of each doctor in charge mainly taking into account the degree of efficacy and safety of each patient. Finally, there is a summation of the evaluation of efficacy, safety and utility for each patient.

4. An assessment of the correlation between utility and efficacy, and utility and safety in five double-blind comparative studies on four different products demonstrated that the utility evaluation system is unreliable with poor intra-rater as well as inter-rater reproducibility. This is a cause for concern as new drug applications in Japan are made mainly on the basis of this utility assessment and may be one of the reasons for ethnic differences between Japan and Western countries.

Introduction

The frequency of adverse reactions and the usual daily dosage of drugs, even for the same indications, vary from country to country. This is seen in Figure 4.1 which shows the difference in the frequency of adverse events following the same dosage of an NSAID in Japan, the EC and the USA. These differences, in general, are ascribed to "ethnic" differences and have been a serious hindrance to the mutual acceptance of clinical data.

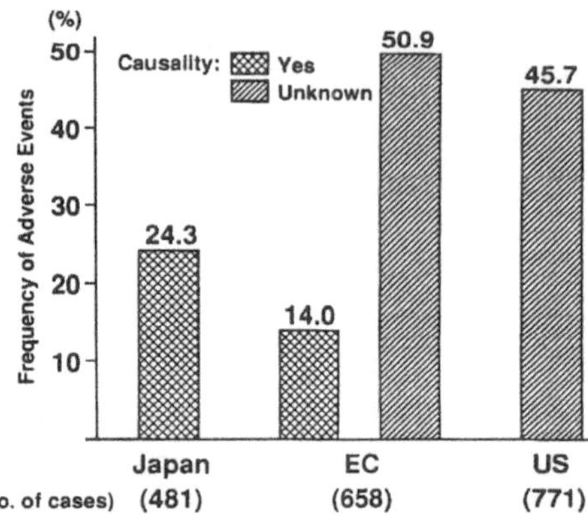

Figure 4.1 Comparison of the frequency of adverse events of an NSAID (20 mg), between Japan, the EC and the USA. (Reproduced from Homma (1992) with permission)

(a) 5-graded evaluation method

Group	Markedly improved (+++)	Moderately improved (++)	Slightly improved (+)	Unchanged (±)	Aggravated (x)	Total No.	Unevaluated
A							

(b) 7-graded evaluation method

Group	Markedly improved (+++)	Moderately improved (++)	Slightly improved (+)	Unchanged (±)	Slightly aggravated (x)	Moderately aggravated (xx)	Markedly aggravated (xxx)	Total No.	Unevaluated
A									

Figure 4.2 Evaluation of efficacy

Ethnic differences in this sense may be caused by genetic and environmental factors. The environmental determinants consist of several factors, including medical custom, philosophy of doctors with respect to drug treatment, doctors' and/or patients' education, doctor–patient inter-relationship, diet, religion and climate etc. In addition, the method of assessing data from clinical studies also seems to be one of the major factors causing so-called ethnic differences in clinical responsiveness following the administration of medicines.

In Japan, some specific evaluation methods have been used for a long period of time and have been a major influence on the new drug approval process in spite of the poor scientific background to this methodology.

Clinical assessment

When investigators in Japan assess new medicines by conducting double-blind comparative or controlled clinical studies, they evaluate efficacy, safety and *yuyosei* in Japanese which is translated into English as utility or usefulness, for each patient. Efficacy is evaluated in terms of improvement by rating it as marked, moderate, slight, unchanged or aggravated (Figure 4.2). Safety is assessed in terms of the degree of adverse events, rated as no problem, slightly problematic, problematic, and seriously problematic, corresponding to no adverse events, the necessity of reducing dosage due to adverse events, the necessity of special treatment for adverse events, and the necessity of stopping medication, respectively (Figure 4.3).

The *yuyosei* or utility for each patient is evaluated by the subjective impression of each doctor-in-charge, mainly taking account of the degree of efficacy and safety of each patient. This utility is usually classified as very useful, moderately useful, slightly useful, not necessarily useful or undetermined, and not useful or harmful (Figure 4.4). This assessment is subjective and depends on the doctor's impression.

Finally, there is a summation of the evaluations of efficacy, safety and utility for each patient. Moreover, it is common for the evaluation of the medicine for a new drug approval to be made on the basis of the utility assessment, rather than the separate assessments of efficacy and/or safety. However, I believe that this "utility" evaluation system is not scientific because of poor intra-rater as well as inter-rater reproducibility.

When a patient is markedly improved without any adverse events, almost all doctors usually judge the product as "very useful".

Group	No problem (–)	Slightly problematic (x)	Problematic (xx)	Seriously problematic (xxx)
A				

Figure 4.3 Evaluation of safety

Key:

No problem: no adverse affects

Slightly problematic:
1. necessity of reducing dosage due to adverse events
   or
2. can be continued in the same dosage due to merely slight adverse events

Problematic: necessity of special treatment for adverse events but medication is continued with or without reducing dosage

Seriously problematic: necessity of stopping medication

Group	Very useful (+++)	Moderately useful (++)	Slightly useful (x)	Undetermined or not necessarily useful (±)	Not useful or harmful (x)
A					

Figure 4.4 Evaluation of utility

However, if a patient is markedly improved but with some adverse events, say headache, some doctors may still rate the assessment as "very useful", but others as "moderately useful" or even "slightly useful", depending on the degree of headache which the doctor perceives. Therefore, the summation of these "utility" results are greatly influenced by the group of doctors carrying out the clinical studies. A distribution of utility evaluations on the basis of the evaluation of efficacy and safety in a double-blind clinical study of an antihypertensive drug are shown in Figure 4.5.

When efficacy was assessed as marked and there were no adverse events, about 82% were evaluated as "very useful", and 18% as "moderately useful". When the efficacy was moderate and there were no problems in safety, about 13% were evaluated as "very

<table>
<tr><td rowspan="3"></td><td rowspan="3"></td><td colspan="20">Safety Rating</td><td rowspan="2">Total
(No.of
cases)</td></tr>
<tr><td colspan="5">No problem</td><td colspan="5">slightly problematic</td><td colspan="5">Problematic</td><td colspan="5">Seriously problematic</td></tr>
<tr><td colspan="5">utility</td><td colspan="5">utility</td><td colspan="5">utility</td><td colspan="5">utility</td><td></td></tr>
<tr><td rowspan="10" style="writing-mode:vertical-lr">Efficacy in terms of Improvement Rating</td><td rowspan="2">Markedly improved</td><td>†††</td><td>††</td><td>†</td><td>±</td><td>−</td><td>†††</td><td>††</td><td>†</td><td>±</td><td>−</td><td>†††</td><td>††</td><td>†</td><td>±</td><td>−</td><td>†††</td><td>††</td><td>†</td><td>±</td><td>−</td><td rowspan="2">80</td></tr>
<tr><td>59
(81.9)</td><td>13
(18.1)</td><td></td><td></td><td></td><td>1
(12.5)</td><td>7
(87.5)</td><td></td><td></td><td></td><td></td><td></td><td></td><td></td><td></td><td></td><td></td><td></td><td></td><td></td></tr>
<tr><td></td><td colspan="5">72</td><td colspan="5">8</td><td colspan="5">0</td><td colspan="5">0</td><td></td></tr>
<tr><td rowspan="2">Moderately improved</td><td>†††</td><td>††</td><td>†</td><td>±</td><td>−</td><td>†††</td><td>††</td><td>†</td><td>±</td><td>−</td><td>†††</td><td>††</td><td>†</td><td>±</td><td>−</td><td>†††</td><td>††</td><td>†</td><td>±</td><td>−</td><td rowspan="2">48</td></tr>
<tr><td>5
(13.2)</td><td>33
(86.8)</td><td></td><td></td><td></td><td></td><td>6
(75)</td><td>2
(25)</td><td></td><td></td><td></td><td></td><td></td><td>2
(100)</td><td></td><td></td><td></td><td></td><td></td><td></td></tr>
<tr><td></td><td colspan="5">38</td><td colspan="5">8</td><td colspan="5">2</td><td colspan="5">0</td><td></td></tr>
<tr><td rowspan="2">Slightly improved</td><td>†††</td><td>††</td><td>†</td><td>±</td><td>−</td><td>†††</td><td>††</td><td>†</td><td>±</td><td>−</td><td>†††</td><td>††</td><td>†</td><td>±</td><td>−</td><td>†††</td><td>††</td><td>†</td><td>±</td><td>−</td><td rowspan="2">42</td></tr>
<tr><td></td><td>18
(46.1)</td><td>20
(51.3)</td><td>1
(25.6)</td><td></td><td></td><td></td><td>2
(100)</td><td></td><td></td><td></td><td></td><td></td><td></td><td></td><td></td><td></td><td></td><td>1
(100)</td><td></td></tr>
<tr><td></td><td colspan="5">39</td><td colspan="5">2</td><td colspan="5">0</td><td colspan="5">1</td><td></td></tr>
<tr><td rowspan="2">Unchanged (Ineffective)</td><td>†††</td><td>††</td><td>†</td><td>±</td><td>−</td><td>†††</td><td>††</td><td>†</td><td>±</td><td>−</td><td>†††</td><td>††</td><td>†</td><td>±</td><td>−</td><td>†††</td><td>††</td><td>†</td><td>±</td><td>−</td><td rowspan="2">19</td></tr>
<tr><td></td><td></td><td>5
(33.3)</td><td>10
(66.7)</td><td></td><td></td><td></td><td></td><td>4
(100)</td><td></td><td></td><td></td><td></td><td></td><td></td><td></td><td></td><td></td><td></td><td></td></tr>
<tr><td></td><td colspan="5">15</td><td colspan="5">4</td><td colspan="5">0</td><td colspan="5">0</td><td></td></tr>
<tr><td rowspan="2">Aggravated</td><td>†††</td><td>††</td><td>†</td><td>±</td><td>−</td><td>†††</td><td>††</td><td>†</td><td>±</td><td>−</td><td>†††</td><td>††</td><td>†</td><td>±</td><td>−</td><td>†††</td><td>††</td><td>†</td><td>±</td><td>−</td><td rowspan="2">1</td></tr>
<tr><td></td><td></td><td></td><td>1
(100)</td><td></td><td></td><td></td><td></td><td></td><td></td><td></td><td></td><td></td><td></td><td></td><td></td><td></td><td></td><td></td><td></td></tr>
<tr><td></td><td colspan="5">1</td><td colspan="5">0</td><td colspan="5">0</td><td colspan="5">0</td><td></td></tr>
<tr><td colspan="2">Total
(No.of cases)</td><td colspan="5">165</td><td colspan="5">22</td><td colspan="5">2</td><td colspan="5">1</td><td>190</td></tr>
</table>

Key (utility): ††† very useful; †† moderately useful; † slightly useful; ± undetermined; — not useful; ( ) %.

Figure 4.5 Relationship of utility to efficacy and safety in a double-blind, comparative clinical study of an antihypertensive drug. Reproduced from Yamamoto (1991) with permission.

useful" and 87% as "moderately useful". However, even when the product was ineffective, if there were no adverse events, some 33% were evaluated as "slightly useful" while 67% were undetermined. This means that even in the case of the same rating of efficacy and safety, the evaluation of utility is widely variable (Table 4.1). This table shows the correlation between utility and efficacy, and between utility and safety in five double-blind, comparative studies on

Table 4.1 Correlation of utility with efficacy and safety in five double-blind comparative clinical studies of various kinds of drugs

Trials		No. of cases	Correlation between efficacy (improvement rating) and utility				Correlation between safety rating and utility			
			Spearman rank correlation coefficient	*Accord- ance rate (%)*	*Discordance rate (%)*		*Spearman rank correlation coefficient*	*Accord- ance rate (%)*	*Discordance rate (%)*	
					One grade	*Two grade and more*			*One grade*	*Two grade and more*
I	Antihypertensive	190	0.75	71.1	27.9	1.1	0.80	70.5	23.2	6.3
II	Antihypertensive	331	0.89	77.1	20.9	2.1	0.45	58.9	27.2	13.9
III	Antipsychotic	93	0.99	86.0	14.0	—	0.94	40.9	48.4	10.8
IV	Antiarrhythmic	103	0.97	88.4	10.7	1.0	0.43	43.7	26.2	30.1
V	Transfusion	100	0.85	80.0	20.0	—	0.79	66.0	32.0	2.0

Adapted from Yamamoto (1991).

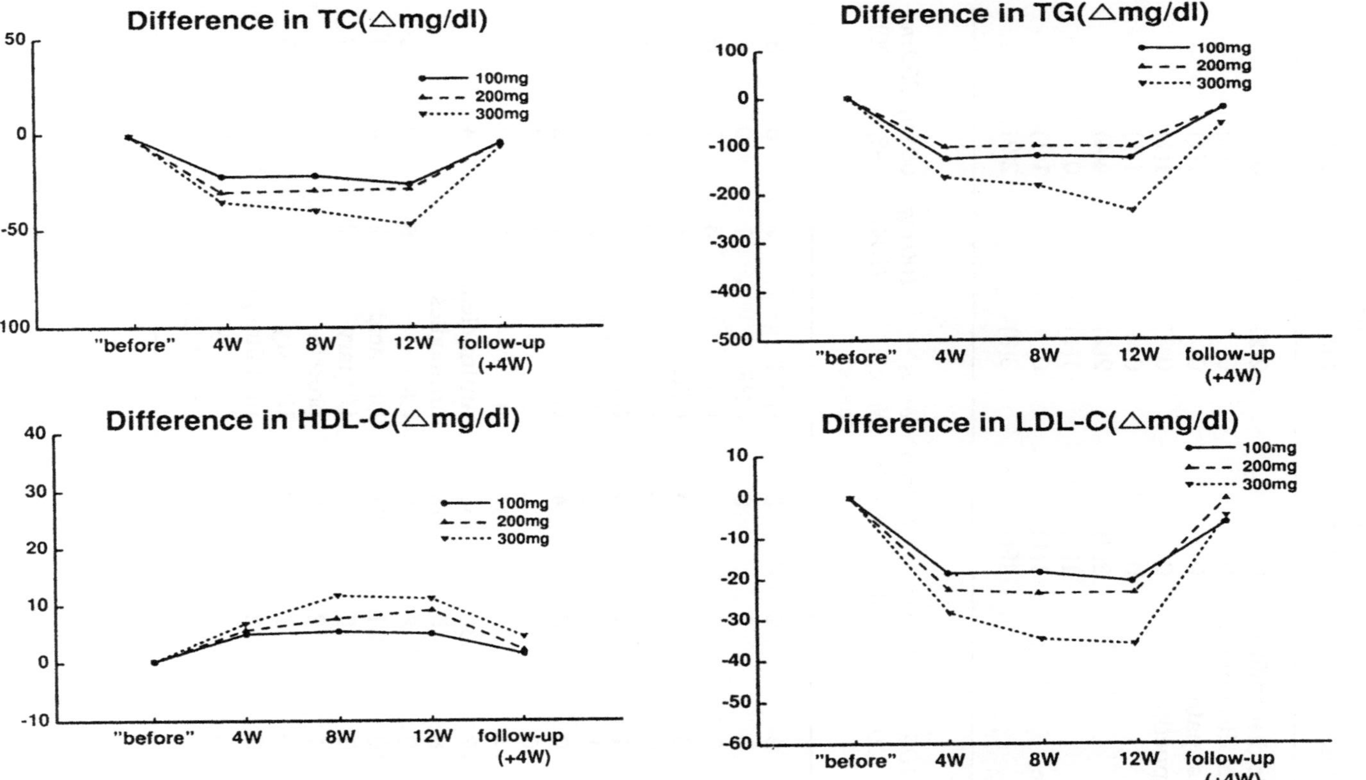

Figure 4.6 Dose-response curve of an antihyperlipidemic drug L. (parallel, double-blind study). TC=total cholesterol, TG=triglyceride, LDL-C=low density lipoprotein cholesterol, HDL-C=high density lipoprotein cholesterol

Table 4.2 Incidence of adverse events observed in the dose-finding study of an antihyperlipidemic drug L. (parallel double-blind study) ( ): %

Items (No. of cases)	100 mg (104)	200 mg (98)	300 mg (109)
Epigastric discomfort	0	2(2)	0
Abdominal discomfort	0	0	1(1)
Abdominal pain	0	0	1(1)
Loss of appetite	0	0	1(1)
Nausea	0	0	1(1)
Eruption	3(3)	2(2)	4(4)
Itching	1(1)	1(1)	0
Lassitude	1(1)	0	1(1)
Others	4(4)	3(3)	2(2)

Items (No. of cases)	100 mg (104)	200 mg (98)	300 mg (109)	Items (No. of cases)	100 mg (104)	200 mg (98)	300 mg (109)
WBC	2	2	3	BUN	7	3	8
RBC	0	2	3	CRE	1	0	6
Hb	0	2	2	UA	3	2	6
Ht	0	3	3	CPK	8	8	8
PLT	0	1	0	FBS	2	1	4
St	1	1	0	Na	0	0	1
Mon	1	0	0	K	4	7	6
Eos	0	3	4	Cl	1	2	2
Bas	0	0	2	Ca	4	4	5
GOT	14	26	34	IP	0	0	1
GPT	17	30	35	Antinuclear antibodies	7	4	4
LDH	8	5	13				
ALP	8	8	9	CRP	5	3	2
rGTP	10	21	28	Uric acid	2	4	3
ChE	1	5	2	Urinary protein	2	2	3
TB	1	2	0				
DB	0	1	0	Urinary urobilinogen	0	1	0
TP	3	3	3				
ALB	0	1	1	Urinary occult blood	3	2	1

Table 4.3 Global safety rating assessed by doctors-in-charge (anti-hyperlipidemic drug L.)

Drug (group)	No problem (–)	Slightly problematic (x)	Problematic (xx)	Seriously problematic (xxx)	Total (No. of cases)
100 mg	75	16	3	10	104
200 mg	61	22	5	10	98
300 mg	61	33	5	10	109
Total (No. of cases)	197	71	13	30	311

Statistical significance test (no protection against multiplicity)

Comparison	p-Value					Meaning
	U-test	Cumul. χ^2	χ^2 (Yates) < x/Total	Fisher	Max t	
100 mg/ 200 mg	0.172	0.403	0.179	0.179	—	no difference
100 mg/ 300 mg	0.034 ($p<5\%$)	0.139	0.021 ($p<5\%$)	0.021 ($p<5\%$)	—	100 mg is safer than 300 mg group
200 mg/ 300 mg	0.504	0.690	0.438	0.438	—	no difference
100 mg/200, 300 mg	—	—	—	—	0.041 ($p<5\%$)	100 mg is safer than 200 mg+300 mg group

four different products. In this comparison the lack of correlation between safety and utility is illustrated by the Spearman's Rank Correlation Coefficients.

The "Accordance Rate" is defined as the relationship between the utility rating which is obtained by subtraction of the safety rating from the efficacy rating. For example, if the efficacy rating is marked (that is point 5) and the safety is no problem (that is point 0), then the utility rating should be "very useful", because point 5 minus point 0 equals point 5, i.e. very useful. Therefore, if the doctor-in-charge evaluated this as "very useful", then that is accordance. However, if the doctor evaluated it as "moderately useful" or "slightly useful" in this case, then this is regarded as discordance. The former is "one grade discordance" and the latter is "two grade discordance". In Table 4.1, both accordance rate and discordance rate varied

Table 4.4 Global improvement rating (efficacy) assessed by doctors-in-charge (antihyperlipidemic drug L.)

Drug (group)	Markedly improved (+++)	Moderately improved (++)	Slightly improved (+)	Unchanged (±)	Aggravated	Total (No. of cases)
100 mg	38	28	22	6	1	95
200 mg	34	25	8	14	1	82
300 mg	57	20	8	6	3	94
Total (No. of cases)	129	73	38	26	5	271

Statistical significance test (no protection against multiplicity)

Comparison	p-Value					Meaning
	U-test	Cumul. χ^2	χ^2 (Yates) >++/Total	Fisher	Max t	
100 mg/ 200 mg	0.912	0.289	0.845	0.847	—	no difference
100 mg/ 300 mg	0.010 (p=1%)	0.023 (p<5%)	0.068 (p<10%)	0.068 (p<10%)	—	300 mg is superior to 100 mg group
200 mg/ 300 mg	0.014 (p<5%)	0.034 (p<5%)	0.164	0.164	—	300 mg is superior to 200 mg group
100, 200 mg/ 300 mg	—	—	—	—	0.0074 (p<0.1%)	300 mg is superior to 100 mg+200 mg group
100 mg/200, 300 mg	—	—	—	—	0.066 (p<10%)	200 mg+300 mg tends to be superior to 100 mg group

widely from study to study. These results clearly indicate that the utility evaluation system is unreliable, even though the author of this paper is one of the proponents for this system (Yamamoto, 1991).

The following are illustrative examples in which the utility evaluation is of no use for the dose finding study. The dose-response of an antihyperlipidemic drug was determined by a parallel, randomised dose–response study with three daily dosage levels of 100 mg, 200 mg and 300 mg. Figure 4.6 shows clearly that 300 mg is the most effective dose and 100 mg is the least effective. Table 4.2 gives details of the

Table 4.5 Utility rating assessed by doctors-in-charge (antihyperlipidemic drug L.)

Drug (group)	Very useful (+++)	Moderately useful (++)	Slightly useful (+)	Undetermined (±)	Not useful	Total (No. of cases)
100 mg	31	32	22	13	1	99
200 mg	26	29	11	19	4	89
300 mg	42	29	14	16	2	103
Total (No. of cases)	99	90	47	48	7	291

Statistical significance test (no protection against multiplicity)

Comparison	p-Value					Meaning
	U-test	Cumul. χ^2	χ^2 (Yates) >++/Total	Fisher	Max $t^{\dagger}$	
100 mg/ 200 mg	0.392	0.190	0.913	0.911	—	no difference
100 mg/ 300 mg	0.330	0.470	0.517	0.518	—	no difference
200 mg/ 300 mg	0.085 ($p<10\%$)	0.169	0.376	0.376	—	almost no difference
100, 200 mg/ 300 mg	—	—	—	—	0.211	no difference

†Max $t = t$ (100, 200/300) = 1.552 $p=0.211$
Max $t = t$ (100, 200/300) = 0.123

adverse events observed. The incidence of some adverse events seems to be slightly higher following 300 mg than after 100 and 200 mg. When these safety data were examined semi-quantitatively by means of the above-mentioned categorised scale (Table 4.3), the incidence of adverse events following 300 mg tended to be higher than that of 100 mg at 5% significance level. If these results are considered, we may choose 300 mg as the optimal dose. However, the utility also has to be assessed. To do so, the quantitative data of efficacy has to be transformed into semi-quantitative data and even here using the semi-quantitatively categorised scale, 300 mg showed the highest efficacy (Table 4.4). Then, each doctor-in-charge evaluates the utility rating for each patient, mainly by taking account of efficacy and safety. The utility results were calculated by summing each utility rating, and here no significant difference was observed among these three dose levels (Table 4.5).

Table 4.6 Several problems inherent to utility evaluation

I.   Scientific aspects
(1) Ambiguous definition:
poor reproducibility (intra-rater as well as inter-rater).
(2) Subjective judgement:
Poor objectivity causes diversity in utility evaluation even for the same efficacy and safety.
(3) Uncertainty in evaluation of safety due to small sample size for real assessment of adverse events.
(4) Utility rating value is of no use for daily medical practice.
(5) Loss of information:
In order to assess "utility", quantitative efficacy data must be transformed into semi-quantitative categorised scale value.

II. Regulatory aspects
(1) Difficulty in discernment between conscientious and fraudulent judgement.
(2) Tendency to develop safer drugs and/or dosages.

Therefore, I believe that in essence the utility evaluation system has many problems and drawbacks from the standpoint of the new drug evaluation, as shown in Table 4.6.

From the scientific viewpoint, the definition of utility is very ambiguous. Usually doctors assess utility mainly by taking account of efficacy and safety, but some doctors insist that the utility should be evaluated from the standpoint of clinical as well as social usefulness. Here they consider not only efficacy and safety but also aspects such as taste, colour, size of tablet and so on, when they evaluate the utility rating. Evaluation of utility varies from doctor to doctor even for the same efficacy rating and the same safety rating. Usually the sample size for Phase III clinical studies is selected to assess mainly efficacy but not safety. However, the sample size is too small to evaluate the safety extensively. It is often difficult to judge some adverse events as to whether they are drug-related adverse reactions or just chance occurrences. It is often difficult to judge whether some adverse events are drug-related or just chance occurences, as when the numbers are small, the distribution can be uneven purely by chance (Pocock, 1983). As the number of apparent adverse events in Phase III clinical studies is not usually large, the judgement of utility could be significantly biased just by chance.

Figure 4.7 shows the safety evaluation results of 125 placebo-controlled double-blind clinical studies. In some studies, the active

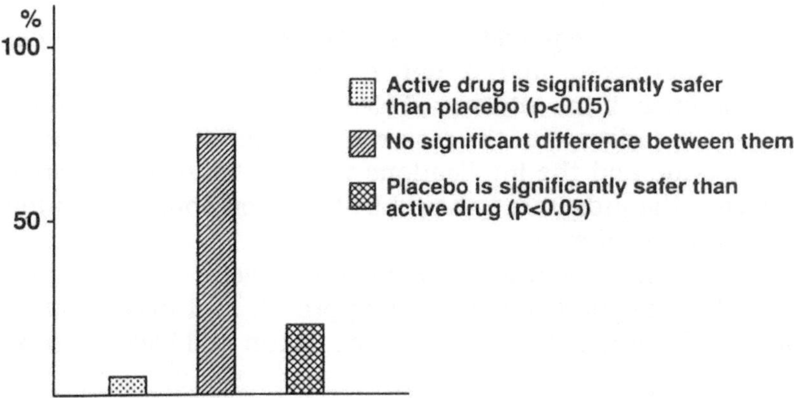

Figure 4.7 Comparison of safety rating between placebos and active drugs in 125 double-blind, placebo-controlled clinical studies

drug was significantly safer that the placebo, but this may be a reflection of uneven distribution of chance occurrences.

In addition to the problems discussed, new drug approvals on the basis of utility tend to lead the pharmaceutical companies to prefer safer drugs to more effective ones. This tendency is in accordance with the Japanese preference in medical practice. Patients as well as doctors in Japan are inclined to choose safer drugs or lower dosages than more effective drugs or higher dosages. This tendency may be supported, at least partly, by the national health insurance system, where patients are not so much concerned about medical fees or economical problems.

Moreover, from the regulatory aspect, an on-site inspector cannot distinguish whether the utility rating results are based on a real conscientious judgement or some fraudulent judgement, because the utility rating is completely dependent on the doctor's subjective impression (Table 4.6).

Conclusions

In conclusion, to date the utility evaluation system is still supported by many clinicians and some biostatisticians. Proponents for the utility system insist that the drug evaluation for new drug approval should be based on the impression of the doctors in the daily medical practice. However, I believe that this concept and attitude has arisen from a misunderstanding and confusion of private or micro level with national or macro level practice. In the private or micro level practice, if the doctor makes a mistake in his or her judgement, the responsibility and the consequences are confined only to that doctor and/or patient. However, in national or macro level practice, if the Ministry of Health and Welfare (MHW) makes a mistake in judgement, the responsibility and the consequences are nation-wide and the implications will be significant. Therefore, in this case the judgement should be based on sound scientific principles and results.

The utility evaluation system has several inherent problems from the viewpoint of new drug approval, and may be one of the causes of ethnic differences between Japan and Western countries.

Acknowledgement

The author greatly appreciates the valuable advice and useful comments of Mr T. Mitsuishi and Mr T. Kurokawa.

References

Homma M (1992). Requirements for assessment of clinical safety regulatory perspectives. In: D'Arcy PF and Harron DWG (eds) *Proceedings of The First International Conference on Harmonisation, Brussels, 1991*. The Queen's University of Belfast, pp. 390–399.

Pocock SJ (1983). *Clinical Trials. A Practical Approach*. John Wiley & Sons, Chichester, p. 75.

Yamamoto K (1991). Utility of drugs and its assessments in clinical trials. *Clin Eval*, **19**:205–212 (in Japanese).

5
The top 50 drugs in the UK and Japan: why are they so different?

KAZUNORI HIROKAWA, COLIN T DOLLERY

Summary

1. This study identified the top 50 drugs according to sales figures (IMS) in Japan and the UK and reviewed the references for clinical trials in Japan in order to determine the factors contributing to the differences in these two groups of medicines.

2. The basic design of the trials reviewed was of a good standard and all were controlled, randomised and double-blind. Only seven of the 55 trials used placebos as controls and 30 out of 44 trials, which used active drugs as controls, failed to show a statistically significant difference in efficacy. Most of the trials were of a substantial size but the number of centres included was large and consequently each centre had only a few patients.

3. Almost all of the trials reviewed used multiple endpoints, but for most drugs these were not fully defined. A unique feature of Japanese studies is the universal use of global response criteria for efficacy although the indices and the methods used to calculate them were rarely fully defined in the published papers.

Introduction

Japan and the UK are both developed countries with clean water, good food hygiene, high standard of living, highly developed medical services and a substantial, innovative, domestic pharmaceutical industry. Mortality from infectious diseases is low in both countries and the predominant causes of death are cardiovascular disease and cancer. One important difference is that coronary heart disease is much more prevalent in the UK than Japan and there are also some differences in the prevalence of some common cancers.[1,2] Both countries share the problem of an ageing population. These characteristics suggest that the amounts of drugs used, in broad pharmacological classes, would be similar even if the particular members of a class reflected local innovation and the marketing strength of domestic pharmaceutical companies. However, superficial examination of the leading drugs, by sales volume, in the two countries showed major differences for which there was no obvious explanation.[3-6] This study of the top 50 drugs in the two countries in 1991 was undertaken to document the differences and try to understand them in terms of clinical trial methodology and local circumstances.

Methods

Drugs in the top 50 in Japan and the UK

The first step in the study was to obtain data published by International Medical Statistics Ltd and to compile a list of the top 50 drugs, by sales volume in Japan (yen) and in the UK (pounds) for the year 1991.[3-6] The drugs are listed in Tables 5.1 and 5.2. Inspection of the tables showed a number of differences, indeed only 12 drugs appear in both tables and 22 drugs in the top 50 in Japan are not even marketed in the UK. We decided at that point to concentrate on the top 50 drugs in Japan to try to understand what factors might have contributed to the observed differences.

Collection of the references describing outcome trials in Japan

Most of the drugs we selected for specific review are not marketed outside Japan and almost all papers about them are in Japanese language publications. This meant that only two references[23,59] could be retrieved through international databases such as "Medline". To obtain publications describing randomised controlled clinical trials about the drugs under study we approached a number of clinicians in Japan who used information sources available in their hospital including literature requested from pharmaceutical company representatives. The publications selected for analysis are not intended to be a comprehensive account of individual drugs but they represent a sample of the largest and best designed studies on them which are available to Japanese physicians.

Other references concerning standard criteria used for evaluation of drug responses in particular disease entities in Japan were also consulted.

Table 5.1 The top 50 drugs in the UK

No.	Product	Generic name	Classification
1.	Zantac	Ranitidine	H_2-blockers
2.	Adalat	Nifedipine	Ca-blockers
3.	Ventolin	Salbutamol	Bronchodilators
4.	Voltarol	Diclofenac	NSAIDs
5.	Becotide	Beclomethasone dipropionate	Steroids inhalers
6.	Becloforte	Beclomethasone dipropionate	Steroids inhalers
7.	Tagamet	Cimetidine	H_2-blockers
8.	Capoten	Captopril	ACE inhibitors
9.	Innovace	Enalapril	ACE inhibitors
10.	Amoxil	Amoxycillin	Penicillins
11.	Zovirax	Acyclovir	Antivirals
12.	Losec	Omeprasole	Proton pump inhibitors
13.	Tenomin	Atenolol	β-blockers
14.	Frumil	Amiloride + frusemide	Diuretics
15.	Sandimmun	Cyclosporin A	Immunosuppressants
16.	Cimetidine	Cimetidine	H_2-blocker
17.	Atenolol	Atenolol	β-blockers
18.	Augmentin	Co-amoxiclav	Penicillins
19.	Gaviscon	Al- & Mg-containing antacids	Antacids

Table 5.1 continued

20.	Minocin	Minocycline	Tetracyclines
21.	Triludan	Terfenadine	Antihistamines
22.	Ciproxin	Ciprofloxacin	New quinolones
23.	Tenoretic	Atenolol + clorthiazide	Antihypertensives
24.	Prozac	Fluoxentine	Antidepressants
25.	Oruvail	Ketoprofen	NSAIDs
26.	Pulmicort	Budesonide	Steroids inhalers
27.	Atrovent	Ipratropium	Bronchodilators
28.	Genotropin	Somatropin	Growth hormones
29.	Prempak-C	Conjugated oestrogens	Sex hormones
30.	Naprosyn	Naproxen	NSAIDs
31.	Timoptol	Timolol	β-blockers
32.	Serevent	Salmeterol	Bronchodilators
33.	Intal	Cromoglycate	Prophylaxis of allergy
34.	Feldene	Piroxicam	NSAIDs
35.	Erythroped	Erythromycin	Macrolides
36.	Canesten	Clotrimazole	Genital antifungals
37.	Beconase	Beclomethasone dipropionate	Nasal aerosol
38.	Marvelon	Ethinyl oestradiol	Oral contraceptives
39.	Epilim	Valproate sodium	Antiepileptics
40.	Amoxycillin	Amoxycillin	Penicillins
41.	Prothiaden	Dothiepin	Antidepressants
42.	Lactulose	Lactulose	Osmotic laxatives
43.	Brufen	Ibuprofen	NSAIDs
44.	Becodisks	Beclomethasone dipropionate	Steroids inhalers
45.	Zyloric	Allopurinol	Xanthine oxidase inhibitors
46.	Estraderm TTS	Oestradiol	Oestrogen patches
47.	Bricanyl	Terbutaline	Bronchodilators
48.	Diprivan	Propofol	Intravenous anaesthetics
49.	Distaclor	Cefaclor	Cephalosporins
50.	Zestril	Lisinopril	ACE inhibitors

Table 5.2 The top 50 drugs in Japan

No.	Product	Generic name	Classification
1.	Mevalotin	Pravastatin	Hypolipidemics
2.	Adalat	Nifedipine	Ca-blockers
3.	Kefral	Cefaclor	Cephalosporins
4.	UFT	Tegaful + Uracil	Antineoplastic drugs
5.	Gaster	Famotidine	H_2-blockers
6.	Iopamiron	Iopamidor	Non-ionic contrast agents
7.	Avan	Idebenone	Psychoanaleptics
8.	Perdipine	Nicardipine	Ca-blockers
9.	Flumarin	Flomoxef	Cephalosporins
10.	Panaldine	Ticlopidine	Antiplatelet agents
11.	Selbex	Teprenone	Anti-ulcerants
12.	Omnipaque	Iohexol	Non-ionic contrast agents
13.	Renivace	Enalapril	ACE inhibitors
14.	Tarivid	Ofloxacin	New quinolones
15.	Zaditen	Ketotifen	Prophylaxis of allergy
16.	Celtect	Oxatomide	Prophylaxis of allergy
17.	Tagamet	Cimetidine	H_2-blockers
18.	Cefspan	Cefixime	Cephalosporins
19.	Foipan	Camostat	Anti-pancreatitis
20.	Marzulene-S	Azulene + L-glutamine	Anti-ulcerants
21.	Methycobal	Mecobalamin	VB_{12} derivatives
22.	Tienam	Imipenem + Cilastatin	Carbapenems
23.	Elen	Indeloxazine	Psychoanaleptics
24.	Epogin	Epoetin	Erythropoietin
25.	Pansporin	Cefotiam	Cephalosporins
26.	Shosaikoto	Shosaikoto	Traditional Chinese medicines
27.	Sermion	Nicergolin	Psychoanaleptics
28.	Loxonin	Loxoprofen	NSAIDs
29.	Tomiron	Cefteram pivoxil	Cephalosporins
30.	Voltaren	Diclofenac	NSAIDs
31.	Captoril	Captopril	ACE inhibitors
32.	Calan	Vinpocetine	Cerebral vasodilators

Table 5.2 continued

33.	Herbesser	Diltiazem	Ca-blockers
34.	Banan	Cefpodoxime proxetil	Cephalosporins
35.	Genotropin	Somatropin	Growth hormones
36.	Alfarol	Alfacalcidol	VD_3 derivatives
37.	Arz	Sodium hyaluronate	Hyaluronic acids
38.	Tenomin	Atenolol	β-blockers
39.	Trildan	Terfenadine	Antihistamines
40.	Celeport	Bifemelane	Psychoanaleptics
41.	Zantac	Ranitidine	H_2-blockers
42.	Baccidal	Norfloxacin	New quinolones
43.	Azeptin	Azelastine	Antihistamines
44.	Cosmocin	Cefuzonac	Cephalosporins
45.	Zovirax	Acyclovir	Antivirals
46.	Elcitonin	Elcatonin	Calcitonins
47.	Intal	Cromoglycate	Prophylaxis of allergy
48.	Frandol	Isosorbide dinitrate	Nitrates
49.	Mohrus	Ketoprofen	NSAIDs (TTS)
50.	Liple	Lipo-alprostadil	Prostaglandins

Review of the references

We reviewed the clinical trial literature available to us, all of which, except one[59], was written in Japanese.[7–58,60–61] This review concentrated on the following factors in Japanese.

(1) Trial design
    (a) Completeness of published description of the protocol.
    (b) Numbers of centres and numbers of patients.
    (c) Randomisation and use of comparison drugs or placebo.
    (d) Duration of study.
    (e) Quality control procedures.

(2) Criteria of response
    (a) Main indices of drug response utilised in the study.
    (b) Validation (e.g. published method) of these indices.
    (c) Use of global response/efficacy scores and adequacy of description of the coefficients or criteria on which they were based.

(d) Statistical analyses used.

Once this had been done a more detailed review was made of a number of individual drugs and categories.

Results

The following account is divided into three sections. The first describes difference in drug use between the two countries, the second deals with general issues concerning clinical trial methodology and the third contains a more detailed analysis of a number of classes of drugs. The analysis concentrated on those drugs which are on the market in Japan but are little used elsewhere. Fifty-five references[7-61] concerning 25 medicines were collected and subjected to detailed review although references to some, e.g. tegaful (anti-cancer, No 4), mecobalamin (vitamin B_{12} derivative, No 21) and Shosaikoto (traditional Chinese medicine, No 26) etc., were not available. Fifty-two of the 55 published references were published between 1980 and 1989, one in 1976 and two in 1979.

Difference in drug use

We compared the drug sales at the exchange rate of 240 yen to the pound sterling since the sales were in 1991. Drug prices were also compared between the two countries.[62-64] The prices of the 28 drugs in the top 50 in Japan, which are also marketed in the UK, differed substantially between the two countries. Terfenadine, ketotifen, oxatomide, atenolol, norfloxacin, somatropin, acyclovir and cromoglycate were all at least twice as expensive in Japan, while the price of diclofenac was half of that in the UK. However, the difference in sales volume cannot be attributed exclusively to the difference in prices.

Total sales of prescription drugs in Japan in 1991 amounted to approximately 26 billion pounds, whereas those in the UK were 3.4 billion pounds.[3-6] Assuming that the population of Japan is roughly twice that of the UK, the Japanese spent 3.8 times as much money on drugs per head of population. According to a report by Japanese Ministry of Health and Welfare, drugs accounted for 30% of total medical expenditure in Japan in 1990,[65] compared with less than 10% in the UK.[66]

Sales of antibiotics in Japan were particularly high at 11 times more than the UK. Sales of cephalosporins were prominent in Japan, whereas the most commonly prescribed antibiotics in the

UK were penicillins. Cefaclor was the most popular cephalosporin in Japan, for example, the sales of which was 29 times as much as that in the UK. In Japan, "psychoanaleptics" or cerebrovasodilators are commonly prescribed to treat senile memory impairment or the sequelae of cerebrovascular diseases but drugs in these categories are scarcely used in the UK.

Vitamins and coenzymes are often prescribed in Japan to relieve symptoms although they are rarely used for this purpose in the UK.

The top selling drug in Japan was pravastatin, an HMG CoA reductase inhibitor. Simvastatin, which is also an HMG CoA reductase inhibitor, did not attain the British top 50, although coronary heart disease is much more prevalent in the UK.

Although several H_2-antagonists are widely used in both countries, drugs whose proposed mechanism of action is to protect the gastric mucosa are widely prescribed in Japan. These drugs, which include teprenone (No 11) and azulene plus L-glutamine (Marzulene-S, No 20), do not inhibit acid secretion or neutralise acid.

Sales of the non-ionic contrast agents, iopamidor (No 6) and iohexol (No 12), were prominent in Japan, while neither of these agents were in the British top 50. A factor in this difference may be efforts in British hospitals to contain costs by limiting the indications for non-ionic contrast agents.

Several anti-allergic agents figure in the top 50 in Japan, whereas only cromoglycate, the first drug of this category, appeared in the top 50 in the UK. Conversely, inhaled steroids and β_2-adrenergic bronchodilators were prominent in the top 50 drugs used in the UK.

Among antiplatelet agents ticlopidine was the No 10 drug in Japan, whereas the drug is not yet on the market in the UK, where aspirin is widely used for similar indications.

Clinical trial methodology

Trial design

Randomisation, blinding and use of placebos: All 55 trials reviewed were randomised, double blind and controlled (Table 5.3). Only seven trials used placebo as a control (Table 5.4). Many physicians in Japan regard all use of placebos as unethical. This creates special difficulties when conclusions are based upon comparisons with established drugs whose efficacy against placebo is poorly validated, e.g. drugs used to treat senile memory impairment.[37–40]

Table 5.3 Summary of design and outcome of clinical trials in Japan

Drug	No. of patients	No. of hospitals	Randomisation	Control	Endpoint	Graded system	Definition of grade	Significance-
Cefaclor	239	26	Yes	CEX	Multiple	Yes	No	N.S.
	310	16	Yes	CEX	Multiple	Yes	Yes	N.S.
	148	12	Yes	CEX	Multiple	Yes	Yes	N.S.
	243	14	Yes	CEX	Multiple	Yes	Yes	N.S.
Cefixime	208	59	Yes	CCL	Multiple	Yes	No	N.S.
	222	59	Yes	AMPC	Multiple	Yes	No	N.S.
	302	32	Yes	CEX	Multiple	Yes	Yes	N.S.
Cefteram-pivoxil	293	52	Yes	CDX	Multiple	Yes	Yes	N.S.
	161	52	Yes	BAPC	Multiple	Yes	No	N.S.
	195	52	Yes	CCL	Multiple	Yes	No	P<0.005
Cefpodoxime-proxetil	186	44	Yes	CCL	Multiple	Yes	No	N.S.
	199	44	Yes	CCL	Multiple	Yes	No	N.S.
	505	59	Yes	CEX	Multiple	Yes	Yes	N.S.
Ofloxacin	279	51	Yes	AMPC	Multiple	Yes	No	N.S.
	250	39	Yes	CCL	Multiple	Yes	No	P<0.001
	262	16	Yes	CCL	Multiple	Yes	No	N.S.
	251	15	Yes	PPA	Multiple	Yes	No	N.S.
	311	23	Yes	PPA	Multiple	Yes	Yes	P<0.001
	320	46	Yes	PPA	Multiple	Yes	Yes	P<0.01
	302	54	Yes	PPA	Multiple	Yes	Yes	N.S.
	258	11	Yes	AMPC	Multiple	Yes	Yes	N.S.
	257	53	Yes	AMPC	Multiple	Yes	Yes	N.S.
Flomoxef	113	30	Yes	LMOX	Multiple	Yes	No	N.S.
	339	64	Yes	LMOX	Multiple	Yes	Yes	N.S.
Imipenem + cilastatin	367	49	Yes	PIPC	Multiple	Yes	No	P<0.05
	289	54	Yes	CPZ	Multiple	Yes	Yes	P<0.01
	151	46	Yes	CZX	Multiple	Yes	Yes	N.S.
Cefotiam	122	39	Yes	CEZ	Multiple	Yes	Yes	P<0.01
	191	28	Yes	CEZ	Multiple	Yes	Yes	N.S.
	146	24	Yes	CEZ	Multiple	Yes	Yes	N.S.
Idebenone	369	61	Yes	Hopantenate	Multiple	Yes	No	N.S.
Indeloxadine	453	93	Yes	Hopantenate	Multiple	Yes	No	P<0.05
Nicergoline	482	141	Yes	Hopantenate	Multiple	Yes	No	N.S.
Bifemelane	379	76	Yes	Hopantenate	Multiple	Yes	No	N.S.
Vinpocetine	383	58	Yes	Ifenprodil	Multiple	Yes	No	N.S.
Teprenone	273	75	Yes	Proglumide	Multiple	Yes	Yes	P<0.05
Azulene + L-glutamine	42	6	Yes	Azulene/L-glu	Multiple	Yes	Yes	N.S.
	80	11	Yes	L-glutamine	Multiple	Yes	Yes	N.S.
Camostat	287	33	Yes	Placebo	Multiple	Yes	No	N.S.
	113	20	Yes	Placebo	Multiple	Yes	No	P<0.01

Table 5.3 continued

Elcatonin	230	28	Yes	Low dose	Multiple	Yes	No/Yes	P<0.01
Alfacalcidol	489	63	Yes	Placebo	Multiple	Yes	No/Yes	P<0.01
Sodium hyaluronate	107	16	Yes	Low dose	Multiple	Yes	No	P<0.01
Loxoprofen	208	8	Yes	Ibuprofen	Multiple	Yes	No	N.S.
	264	36	Yes	Diclofenac	Multiple	Yes	No	N.S.
Epoetin	179	30	Yes	Placebo	Multiple	Yes	No/Yes	P<0.001
Lipo -alprostadil	112	15	Yes	Alprostadil	Multiple	Yes	No/Yes	P<0.05
	138	49	Yes	Alprostadil	Multiple	Yes	No/Yes	P<0.05
Ketotifen	137	35	Yes	Cromoglycate	Multiple	Yes	No/Yes	N.S.
	198	29	Yes	Placebo	Multiple	Yes	No/Yes	N.S.
Pravastatin	284	60	Yes	Clinofibrate	Multiple	Yes	No/Yes	P<0.001
	352	59	Yes	Probucol	Multiple	Yes	No/Yes	P<0.001
	118	18	Yes	Placebo	Multiple	Yes	Yes	P<0.01
Ticlopidine	202	22	Yes	Placebo	Multiple	Yes	No/Yes	P<0.01
	340	101	Yes	Aspirin	Multiple	Yes	No/Yes	P<0.05

Size: Most of the trials were of a substantial size and 60% included over 200 patients (Table 5.5). None described any calculation of the numbers required to detect a stated difference with a given level of statistical significance. Only 21 of the 55 showed a significant difference in efficacy between the two main groups in the trial (Table 5.3). There was an apparent assumption that failure to show a difference could be equated with equal efficacy. The number of centres included in most of the trials was large; in one trial with nicergoline[33] there were 141 centres and 30–50 centres were common place (Table 5.3). Although multi-centre trials are now almost universal in Phase III, because of the difficulty of recruiting adequate numbers from one centre, quality control can become a problem. In the studies we reviewed over one-third of the centres had less than five patients and half had less than ten (Table 5.4). The main quality control procedure appears to have been a meeting of principal investigators but ongoing quality control procedures were rarely described.

Duration: Fifty-two of 55 references reviewed describe the duration of trials. Duration varied from 5 to 22 months, the most frequent being 7–8 months. There seems to be no clear relationship between the duration of the trial and the likely duration of therapeutic use.

Table 5.4 Control used in clinical trials

Control	The number of trials
Active drug	44 (80%)
Placebo	7 (13%)
Low dose of active drug	2 (3.6%)
Constituents	2 (3.6%)
Total	55

Table 5.5 The size of a clinical trial

The number of patients in a trial	The number of trials
<100	2 (3.6%)
–150	10 (18%)
–200	8 (15%)
–250	8 (15%)
–300	5 (9.1%)
–350	8 (15%)
–400	10 (18%)
>400	4 (7.3%)
Total	55

Response criteria

Indices of drug response: Almost all the trials reviewed used multiple endpoints designed to evaluate efficacy, symptoms, adverse reactions etc. (Table 5.3). For three drug categories, the methods used are based on published descriptions with clear endpoints. Urinary tract infections were scored using criteria published by the UTI Committee (Committee on Urinary Tract Infections) in Japan which included grades of pain on micturition, back or lower abdominal pain, neutrophil count in urine, bacterial count in urine, fever etc.[67] Antibiotic responses for skin,[3,22] upper respiratory tract[34] dental,[4] otolaryngal[26,27,36] and gynaecological[28] infections were scored using well defined composite criteria in some trials. Anti-ulcer drugs were studied using standardised gastroscopic criteria.[68] For many other drugs the situation was less satisfactory. Large numbers of endpoints were specified without a clear definition of any of them.

Global response indices: A unique feature of Japanese trials is the use of global response criteria which attempt to reduce conclusions about efficacy and utility to a single number. These figures are reminiscent of the recording of physician and patient preferences in some double-blind trials outside Japan. One of the main reasons for the use of global response indices is that the Japanese Ministry of Health and Welfare recommends such an analysis when a marketing submission for a new drug is made.[69] The composition of the coefficients making up the global responses indices was rarely fully defined. The published papers do not describe what attempts were made to standardise the recording of global response indices.

Statistics: Thirty of 44 trials, which used active drugs as controls, failed to show a statistically significant difference in efficacy (Table 5.3). Often the authors concluded or implied that the test drug was as good as the comparison drug, without any consideration of the type II error inherent in that conclusion.

To most reviewers it might seem unsatisfactory that a new drug had failed to demonstrate superior efficacy to the established agent with which it had been compared. However, this does not seem to be the case in Japan where a trial of this kind can provide a sufficient basis for wide adoption of the new remedy based upon theoretical advantages, derived from preclinical pharmacology, supported by an active marketing campaign. One of the problems of using multiple endpoints is the very large number of statistical comparisons that are possible. Not surprisingly, trials that failed to show important differences in efficacy usually showed some statistically significant differences for some of the many endpoints used. If the trial was stratified, at the time of randomisation sub-group analysis is justified but the scientific validity of multiple *post hoc* analyses is doubtful and they should be regarded as no more than hypothesis generators.

Publication

All of the references except one reviewed were published in Japanese journals. However, it might have been difficult for those papers to be accepted by an international journal, even when translated into English, because of their style and length. Most of the references had about 20 pages and some have more than 40 pages (mean: 24 pages). The reason for this length was the inclusion of lengthy tables of results.

Specifics of some drug categories

We summarise the outcome clinical trials of some drug categories the therapeutic use of which showed prominent differences between the two countries.

Antibiotics

All antibiotics reviewed were compared with active drugs and only seven out of 30 trials showed a statistically significant superiority of the test drug to the comparison agent (Table 5.3). In the other 23 trials the test drug failed to show statistically significant different efficacy from the comparison drug with the implied inference that this meant that it was of equal efficacy. In all trials of urinary tract infections[8,13,14,19,24,25,30,32,35] and one trial in pneumonia[34] antibiotics were evaluated using composite criteria defined clearly in references. For urinary tract infections a number of items were scored separately: e.g. fever, frequency, four grades of pain on micturition, residual urine volume, back or lower abdominal pain, neutrophils in urine and bacteria in urine. For pneumonia a similar list of items for evaluation was provided: fever, cough, dyspnea, chest pain, sputum type and volume, rates, cyanosis, cardiac insufficiency, neutrophil count, ESR and chest radiographic appearance. These items could be scored separately and were also brought into a composite score. Composite criteria for urinary tract infections were universally used since they had been proposed by the UTI Committee in Japan,[67] whereas the criteria for pneumonia proposed by one group of investigators were used only in a trial.[34] Well defined composite criteria were also used to evaluate antibiotic responses for skin,[3,22] dental,[4] otolaryngeal[26,27,36] and gynaecological[28] infections. In the other trials, the criteria used to evaluate drug responses were not fully defined.

Psychoanaleptics and cerebral vasodilators

All of the four psychoanaleptics were compared with hopantenate and only indeloxazine[38] (Elen, No 23) showed a statistically significant difference in efficacy. Hopantenate is on the market in Japan and showed significantly greater efficacy (69%) than an inactive placebo (44%) in an earlier trial in patients with arteriosclerotic and post-stroke memory impairment.[71] In the four trials with psychoanaleptics reviewed in this paper the efficacy rate recorded for hopantenate was almost the same, e.g. 69,[37] 64,[38] 68,[39] and 68%.[40]

Rather than relying upon the earlier trial of hopantenate against placebo it would have been much more convincing to have compared each of the new drugs with a placebo and it is difficult to see any ethical objection to doing so. All the trials with psychoanaleptics used multiple endpoints and were evaluated mainly by using a general improvement index the criteria for which was not fully defined in the references. The number of hospitals involved in a trial was more than 60 and consequently the number of patients evaluated in each hospital was only 3–6.

A cerebral vasodilator vinpocetine (No 32), used for similar indications, was compared with a marketed cerebral vasodilator, ifenprodil, and showed no significant superiority to it[41] while ifenprodil, itself, had shown greater efficacy than a placebo in another trial.[72]

None of these trials can be regarded as providing completely convincing evidence of efficacy for a condition in which the value of drug therapy is still controversial.

Anti-ulcer drugs (mucosal protective agents)

Teprenone (No 11) was compared with proglumide in a randomised double-blinded controlled trial.[42] The endpoint used was gastroscopy with a standardised classification used in Japan which describes the morphology of ulcers.[68] Multiple endpoints were used but the only one that was vigorously defined was the gastroscopic classification. The final clinical effectiveness assessed by gastroscopy shows a significant difference (81.7% improvement for teprenone and 70.1% for proglumide). The only serious criticism of this trial was the use of proglumide as a comparison drug. It might have been better to use a placebo as the response rate for teprenone was comparable to that reported with proglumide in other studies of gastric ulcer healing.[73]

Azulen plus L-glutamine (Marzulene-S, No 20) has had much less extensive testing. The main use of this drug in Japan appears to be in the treatment of drug- or alcohol-induced gastritis. The only randomised control trial we were able to evaluate compared 42 patients of whom 16 were on Marzulene-S, 14 on glutamine alone and 12 on azulene alone.[43] Not surprisingly, given these small numbers, there was no significant difference. The endpoint was endoscopic evaluation of gastric ulcer. There is also a trial report which comparing 80 patients with duodenal ulcer treated with Marzulene-S or L-glutamine which showed no significant difference.[44]

Thus we conclude in the case of Marzulene-S that there is relatively little evidence of efficacy in respect of its main use.

Drugs for osteoporosis or osteoarthritis

Elcatonin (No 46)

This drug is Eel calcitonin produced by chemical synthesis. Its main use is the treatment of pain in patients with osteoporosis. The trial reviewed was a study of 230 patients half of whom received a full dose and half a quarter of that dose.[47] There was no placebo control. The main index of response was lumbosacral pain assessed by patient evaluation on a four point scale (the scale ran from severe pain, bad pain, mild pain to no pain). The drug was given over four weeks twice a week; 67.6% of patients treated with Eel calcitonin showed improvement on the full dose versus 48.4% of patients on the reduced dose. A weakness of the design was the relatively short period of treatment for a chronic condition and the decision to use a reduced dose rather than a placebo as the comparator.

Alfacalcidol (No 36)

This drug is a derivative of vitamin D (1α-OH-D_3). The study was placebo controlled and double blind. The endpoints used included changes in bone pain graded by using a visual analogue scale, microdensitometry of bone radiographs and "general improvement rate", the scoring of which was not defined in the description.[48] The general improvement rate in the alfacalcidol group was superior to that in the placebo group, showing statistically significant difference by the Mann–Whitney U-Test. More importantly, this drug relieved bone pain and inhibited the decrease in bone density significantly compared with placebo.

Sodium hyaluronate (No 27)

Sodium hyaluronate, extracted from cockscombs and purified, is given by intra-articular injection to relieve arthritic pain in osteoarthritis. The drug is believed to function as an articular lubricant and ameliorate the degeneration of cartilage. In the trial reviewed the "general improvement rate" with sodium hyaluronate (0.5% solution) was 60.4% and that with the control (0.01% solution of the drug) was 34.0%, showing a significant difference although the method used to derive the rating of improvement was not clearly defined.[49] Overall there was no effect upon pain at rest but a significant improvement in pain while walking or climbing stairs. The composite score used was not described in sufficient detail to be evaluable.

Loxoprofen (No 28)

Loxoprofen is the top selling NSAID in Japan with the claim that its anti-inflammatory action is 20 times and 10 times greater than that of indomethacin and ketoprofen respectively, on a weight basis. It is claimed to be a less irritant drug to gastric mucosa than other NSAIDs. The clinical efficacy of the drug was studied in lumbago or osteoarthritis compared with ibuprofen[50] or diclofenac.[51] The method of grading the response was not fully defined in either trial. Neither trial demonstrated superior efficacy of loxoprofen to the comparison drug. No significant difference was observed in the frequency of adverse reactions although animal studies had suggested a higher therapeutic index with loxoprofen.

Drugs with a readily measurable effect

Epoetin (No 24)

This drug is human erythropoietin produced by recombinant DNA technology. As expected, the drug increased haemoglobin in patients with chronic renal failure significantly compared with placebo after eight weeks' treatment.[52] It also decreased the number of patients receiving a transfusion, the frequency of transfusion and the amount of blood transfused, significantly. Despite this clearcut endpoint "general efficacy" was also evaluated using an arbitrary grading.

Pravastatin (No 1)

Although the effect of this drug on serum cholesterol level was clear and substantial, efficacy was also evaluated based on arbitrary, "global efficacy" criteria in two of three trials.[57–59] It is interesting to note that the drug was compared with clinofibrate[57] and probucol[58] in two trials and with placebo in only one.[59]

Discussion

Total sales of prescription drugs in Japan are about eight times larger than in the United Kingdom although the population is only just over twice as large.[3-6] Drug expenditure in Japan represents almost 30% of healthcare expenditure[65] compared with about 10% in the UK.[66] There are also major differences in the types of drug in widespread use. Comparing the top 50 drugs by sales volume in the two countries, only 12 appeared on both lists (Tables 5.1, 5.2). Differences in drug utilisation based on the country of original discovery and the relative marketing strengths of domestic and foreign producers would be anticipated but 22 drugs in the Japanese top 50 are not on the market in the UK at all.[63] Part of the reason for these differences lies in the processes of drug evaluation and part in the method of remuneration.

The basic design of the trials reviewed was of a good standard and all were controlled, randomised and double blind (Table 5.3). The control group rarely involved the use of a placebo and was usually a comparison with a standard drug or with a lower dose of the same one. In therapeutic areas, such as infections where placebos cannot be used for ethical reasons, this design is unavoidable. However, in other areas such as drugs used to treat senility, arthritis, osteoporosis etc., it would have been more informative if placebos had been used in some of the trials. A particular problem was comparison with another "active" drug whose efficacy had itself not been fully established, e.g. hopantenate as the comparator in trials of psychoanaleptics.[37-40]

A further feature of the Japanese trials was the very large number of participating centres, up to 141 in one case and 35 to 50 centres in others (Table 5.3). This is partly a consequence of many pharmaceutical companies trying to develop similar compounds in a limited number of recognised centres, mainly universities and associated hospitals. The number of respected investigators is also limited and companies wish these investigators to participate in their studies because of the authority this gives to the data. For example, in the studies of different psychoanaleptics the authors list shows many names in common.[37-40]

To an outsider the large number of centres must pose serious problems in achieving uniform application of the protocols, particularly when some of the response criteria are not fully defined. To maintain data quality it is normal practice in Japan for the principal investigators to meet before the study begins and at intervals during it. The junior doctors, who usually carry out the day to day work required by the study do not usually participate in these conferences (although this is a problem which also occurs elsewhere in the world). During the study pharmaceutical company personnel visit the participating centres and maintain contact with the investigators. The conduct of clinical trials has been regulated by a Japanese code of good clinical practice (GCP) since 1990.[74]

A striking feature of the trial protocols was the use of multiple endpoints and of global indices of response. In some instances (e.g. urinary tract infections) the endpoints were clearly defined but in many the lengthy published papers gave insufficient details to fully evaluate the methodology. Often responses were graded as "excellent", "good", "fair", "poor" etc. To the clinician this classification may have been sensible and obvious but to a reviewer, particularly from another country, it is almost impossible to know what the criteria mean and whether or not they have been uniformly applied.

The use of global indices of efficacy, usefulness etc., was almost universal even for drugs such as epoetin (erythropoietin)[52] or pravastatin (HMG CoA reductase inhibitor)[57,58] where the rise in haemoglobin or fall in total cholesterol seems to be sufficient evidence in itself. The use of these indices is recommended by the Japanese Ministry of Health and Welfare in its guidelines.[65] The concept of trying to reach a conclusion about the overall value of a drug is clearly a useful one, but the lack of any definition of the index in most studies makes it very difficult for an outsider to interpret it. For example, it is not clear at what stage the factors to be taken into account in assessing global response are defined. In many cases the index appears to be a global impression reached by the investigator rather than a formally defined parameter.

The majority of the trials reviewed failed to show any significant difference between the new drug and the established agent with which it was compared (Table 5.3). In most countries failure to demonstrate a clinical advantage in efficacy terms would limit acceptance of a new product but this does not appear to be so much the case in Japan. A negative trial is interpreted as meaning that the new drug has the same efficacy as the old one without the power of the trial to quantify a negative conclusion being taken into account. If the new drug has some theoretical advantages and appears to be at least as efficacious, and most importantly as safe, as the old one this seems to be sufficient to provide a basis for marketing.

One of the main reasons for this unusual state of affairs probably lies in the nature of the drug market in Japan and the pressures on the industry to innovate. General practitioners in Japan often dispense their own medicines and an important part of their income is derived from the difference between wholesale and retail prices of the agents they prescribe. Most hospitals have no general budget for drugs because they form part of the recharge to the patient's insurance and the hospitals also gain from the mark-up on the drugs their staff have prescribed. This situation is beginning to change and the government has prohibited hospitals from negotiating prices individually with pharmaceutical representatives.

The Japanese Government has brought pressure on the pharmaceutical companies by a programme of reducing prices every two years. In the case of some antibiotics the reduction is of the order of 20%, but for most other drugs the reduction is closer to 10%. A newly introduced drug, which is judged more effective (based on preclinical and clinical data) may command a higher price than an established agent. Thus, companies are under exceptional pressure to introduce new compounds at regular intervals to maintain their income. Obviously, this programme has encouraged Japanese pharmaceutical companies to develop new compounds although many of them have relatively minor differences from established ones.

Another feature of Japanese medicines, especially of antibiotics, are wide indications. New, potent, broad spectrum antibiotics are studied in patients with common infections to obtain approval for wide indications. Serious problems with multiple-resistant staphylococcal infections in Japanese hospitals may be partly caused by prescription of powerful antibiotics with a broad spectrum for relatively minor infections.

Several other factors are also important to elucidate the difference in drug use between the two countries, e.g. nationality, genetic differences, economic, social and cultural variations. Apart from a traditional preference for medicines in Japan, the possibility of genetic differences in sensitivity to drugs should be taken seriously. Widespread prescription of anti-ulcer drugs has been explained by hypothesising that the gastric mucosa of Japanese is more sensitive to irritants. Hence Japanese physicians co-prescribe anti-ulcer drugs with other medicines. There are so far to our knowledge, few clinical trials addressing genetic differences in drug response between Europeans and Japanese although pharmacokinetic differences have been widely studied.

The criteria for the approval of medicines by government agencies differ from one country to another and these differences are an obstacle to rapid and economical international development and marketing. Recently, however, efforts have been made to harmonise the criteria between countries, resulting in the First International Conference on Harmonisation held in Brussels in 1991. Japan is one of the most important world markets for therapeutic drugs and has already launched several promising, innovative, medicines into the world market. However, the very different approach to clinical trial design and analysis adopted in Japan is a barrier to international acceptance of data about products developed in that country. Among the features which cause difficulty are reluctance to use placebos, a multiplicity of endpoints, large numbers of centres (each with few patients) without well defined quality control procedures and use of global response and utility ratings which are not clearly defined. On the positive side almost all the trials reviewed were controlled, randomised and double blind and contained substantial numbers of patients. Improvements of clinical trial methodology can be anticipated since new "Guidelines on statistical analyses in clinical trials" and "General guidelines on clinical evaluation of new drugs" were published in 1992.[75,76] Improvements recommended in the guidelines include determination of the size of a trial with consideration of type I and II statistical errors, defining a single primary endpoint, if possible, to avoid abuse of statistics and the limiting number of centres included in a trial to maintain data quality. Given that background it should not be too difficult for Japanese investigators and their sponsors to bring their clinical trial methodology into closer conformity with the approaches used in Europe and North America.

Acknowledgement

We thank Mr David Brown and Ms Samantha Gurnah of International Medical Statistics for permission to use data on the most widely prescribed drugs in the United Kingdom and Japan.

References

1. Ueie K, Kanai T, Hashimoto Y *et al.* (1992). The general situation of mortality rate in 1990. *Kosei no Shihyo*, **39**(5):22–33 (in Japanese).
2. Office of Population Censuses and Surveys. (1991). Review of the Registrar General on deaths by cause, sex and age, in England and Wales, 1990. In: *Mortality Statistics, Cause.* HMSO, London.
3. *British Hospital Index.* (1991). International Medical Statistics, Ltd., Middlesex.
4. *British Pharmaceutical Index.* (1991). International Medical Statistics, Ltd., Middlesex.
5. Japan Pharmaceutical Market. (1991). IMS Japan, Ltd., Tokyo.

6. *Japan Medical Data Index*. (1991). IMS Japan, Ltd., Tokyo.

7. Matsumoto K, Saito R, Nagahama F *et al.* (1981). A comparative clinical study of cefaclor and cephalexin in bacterial bronchitis. *Chemotherapy (Tokyo)* **29**:653–97 (in Japanese).

8. Ishigami J, Mita T, Ohno S *et al.* (1981). Clinical evaluation of cefaclor in acute simple cystitis. A double-blind comparative study of cefaclor. *Chemotherapy (Tokyo)*, **29**:250–66 (in Japanese).

9. Arata J, Yamamoto Y, Nohara N *et al.* (1981). A double-blind comparison between cefaclor and cephalexin in the treatment of acute bacterial skin infections. *Chemotherapy (Tokyo)*, **29**:267–79 (in Japanese).

10. Horii M, Morinaga T, Takeuchi T *et al.* (1984). A double-blind comparison between cefaclor and cephalexin in the treatment of dental infections. *Jpn J Antibiotics*, **37**:152–75 (in Japanese).

11. Konno K, Saitoh A, Ohizumi K *et al.* (1986). Comparison of cefixime and cefaclor in bacterial bronchitis. *Chemotherapy (Tokyo)*, **34**:1150–83 (in Japanese).

12. Konno K, Saitoh A, Ohizumi K *et al.* (1986). Comparative test of the efficacy of cefixime and amoxicillin on pneumonia by double-blind method. *Chemotherapy (Tokyo)*, **34**:1184–218 (in Japanese).

13. Arakawa S, Fujii A, Kamidono S *et al.* (1986). A double-blind study to compare cefixime and L-cephalexin for the treatment of complicated urinary tract infections. *Nishinippon Hinyoukika*, **48**:645–74 (in Japanese).

14. Kawada Y, Kumamoto E, Nishimoto T *et al.* (1986). Comparative study of T-2588 and cefadroxil in complicated urinary tract infections. *Chemotherapy (Tokyo)*, **34**:908–29 (in Japanese).

15. Kobayashi H, Kawai S, Saitoh A *et al.* (1986). Comparative clinical study of T-2588 and Bacampicillin for bacterial pneumonia by double-blind method. *Kansensyougaku Zasshi*, **60**:1078–106 (in Japanese).

16. Kobayashi H, Kawai S, Saitoh A *et al.* (1986). Comparative clinical study of T-2588 and cefaclor for chronic respiratory tract infections by a double-blind method. *Kansensyougaku Zasshi*, **60**:1052–77 (in Japanese).

17. Shiba K, Saitoh A, Shimada J *et al.* (1988). Comparative clinical study of CS-807 and cefaclor for bacterial pneumonia by a double-blind method. *Kansensyougaku Zasshi*, **62**:973–1001 (in Japanese).

18. Shiba K, Saitoh A, Shimada J *et al.* (1988). Comparative clinical study of CS-807 and cefaclor for chronic respiratory tract infections by a double-blind method. *Kansensyougaku Zasshi*, **62**:1166–91 (in Japanese).

19. Ogata N, Kumazawa J, Kushimoto T *et al.* (1988). A double-blind study to compare CS-807 and L-cephalexin for the treatment of complicated urinary tract infections. *Nishinippon Hinyoukika*, **50**:2077–98 (in Japanese).

20. Kobayashi H, Takamura K, Kono K *et al.* (1984). Comparison of DL-8280 and amoxicillin in the treatment of respiratory tract infection. *Kansensyougaku Zasshi*, **58**:525–54 (in Japanese).
21. Fujimori 1, Kobayashi Y, Obana M *et al.* (1984). Comparative clinical study of ofloxacin and cefaclor in bacterial bronchitis. *Kansensyougaku Zasshi*, **58**:832–61 (in Japanese).
22. Fujita K, Nakano M, Nonami E *et al.* (1984). Comparative clinical study of DL-8280 and cefaclor for suppurative skin and soft tissue infections by a double-blind method. *Kansensyougaku Zasshi*, **58**:793–819 (in Japanese).
23. Saito M, Seo T, Matsubara Y *et al.* (1984). Comparison of clinical efficacy of ofloxacin (OFLX: DL8280) and pipemidic acid (PPA) in acute infectious diarrhoea by a double-blind method. *Kansensyougaku Zasshi*, **58**:965–81 (in Japanese).
24. Kishi H, Nito H, Saitoh I *et al.* (1984). Comparative studies of DL-8280 and pipemidic acid in complicated urinary tract infections by double-blind method. *Hinyoukiyou*, **30**:307–55 (in Japanese).
25. Ishigami J, Kamidono S, Harada M *et al.* (1984). A double-blind controlled study of DL-8280 in comparison with pipemidic acid in the treatment of acute simple cystitis. *Nishinippon Hinyoukika*, **46**:967–88 (in Japanese).
26. Kawamura S, Fukimaki Y, Iwasawa T *et al.* (1984). A comparative double-blind study of DL-8280 and pipemidic acid in suppurative otitis media. *Otologia Fukuoka*, **30**:642–70 (in Japanese).
27. Sasaki T, Unno T, Tomiyama T *et al.* (1984). Evaluation of clinical effectiveness and safety of DL8280 in acute lacunar tonsillitis; in comparison with amoxicillin by double-blind method. *Otologia Fukuoka*, **30**:484–513 (in Japanese).
28. Takase Z, Komoto K, Katayama M *et al.* (1984). Comparative clinical study of ofloxacin (OFLX) and amoxicillin (AMPC) on the infectious disease in the field of obstetrics and gynaecology. *Chemotherapy (Tokyo)*, **34**:31–63 (in Japanese).
29. Ohizumi K, Saitoh A, Nagahama F *et al.* (1987). Comparative double-blind study of the efficacy of 6315-S (Flomoxef) and Latamoxef on chronic respiratory tract infections. *Chemotherapy (Tokyo)*, **35** (Suppl 1):780–809 (in Japanese).
30. Kumazawa J, Matsumoto T, Kumamoto E *et al.* (1987). 6315-S (Flomoxef) in complicated urinary tract infections: a double-blind controlled study using LMOX. *Chemotherapy (Tokyo)*, **35** (Suppl 1):1 138–63 (in Japanese).
31. Soejima R, Matsushima T, Kawane H *et al.* (1986). Comparative study of MK-0787/MK-0791 and piperacillin in respiratory tract infections. *Kansensyougaku Zasshi*, **60**:345–77 (in Japanese).
32. Kawada Y, Nishiura T, Kumamoto E *et al.* (1986). Comparative study of MK-0787/MK-0791 and cefoperazone in complicated urinary tract infections. *Chemotherapy (Tokyo)*, **34**:536–60 (in Japanese).

33. Yura J, Shinagawa N, Ishikawa S *et al.* (1986). Comparative clinical study of imipenem/cilastatin sodium and ceftizoxime in the treatment of purulent peritonitis. *Chemotherapy (Tokyo)*, **34**:713-38 (in Japanese).

34. Matsumoto K, Uzuka Y, Shishido H *et al.* (1979). Clinical evaluation of cefotiam (SCE-963) in pulmonary infections: a comparative study with cefazolin by a randomized double-blind technique. *Chemotherapy (Tokyo)*, **27** (Suppl 3):399–419 (in Japanese).

35. Ishigami J, Ohno S, Tomioka O *et al.* (1979). Clinical evaluation of cefotiam (SCE-963) in complicated urinary tract infections: a comparative study with cefazolin by a randomized double blind technique. *Chemotherapy (Tokyo)*, **27** (Suppl 3):629–48 (in Japanese).

36. Baba S, Iwasawa T, Kawamura S *et al.* (1983). Clinical evaluation of cefotiam (SCE-963) in suppurative otitis media: a comparative study with cefazolin by a randomized double-blind technique. *Jitenn*, Suppl 5:451–68 (in Japanese).

37. Ohtomo E, Araki G, Hasegawa K *et al.* (1985). Clinical efficacy of CV-2619 (Idebenone) in the treatment of cerebrovascular disorders. Multi-centre double-blind study in comparison with Ca-hopantenate. *Igaku no Ayumi*, **134**:220–42 (in Japanese).

38. Ohtomo E, Tohgi H, Hirai S *et al.* (1986). Clinical effectiveness of YM-08054 (Indeloxazine) in the treatment of cerebrovascular disorders. Multi-centre double-blind study in comparison with Ca-hopantenate. *Igaku no Ayumi*, **136**:535–55 (in Japanese).

39. Ohtomo E, Hirai S, Hasegawa K *et al.* (1986). Clinical evaluation of TA-079 (Nicergoline) in the treatment of cerebrovascular disorders. Multi-centre double-blind study in comparison with Ca-hopantenate. *Clin Eval*, **14**:575–602 (in Japanese).

40. Tasaki Y, Kutsuzawa T, Tohgi H *et al.* (1986). Clinical efficacy of E-0687 (Bifemelane) in the treatment of cerebrovascular disorders. Multi-centre double-blind study in comparison with Ca-hopantenate. *Igaku no Ayumi*, **137**:647–70 (in Japanese).

41. Atarashi J, Araki G, Itoh E *et al.* (1983). Clinical efficacy of TCV-3B (Vinpocetin) in the treatment of cerebrovascular disorders. Multi-centre double-blind study in comparison with Ifenprodil tartarate. *Igaku no Ayumi*, 1983;124:66–90 (in Japanese).

42. Serizawa S, Shirakawa K, Sakita T *et al.* (1983). Clinical efficacy of E-0671 (Tetraprenylacetone) in the treatment of gastric ulcer. Multi-centre double-blind study with proglumide. *Prog Med*, **3** (Suppl):1 169–91 (in Japanese).

43. Ichita F, Tashiro N, Murayama H *et al.* (1976). Clinical efficacy of Marzulene-S granule in the treatment of gastric ulcer. Double-blind study with L-glutamine or azulene. *Shinyaku to Rinsho*, **25**:167–75 (in Japanese).

44. Kobayashi S, Sekiguchi T, Takei A *et al.* (1981). Clinical study of Marzulene-S granule in the treatment of duodenal ulcer. Double-blind

study with L-glutamine. *Shinyaku to Rinsho*, **30**:1855–73 (in Japanese).

45. Ishii K, Takebe T, Hirayama N *et al.* (1980). Clinical evaluation of FOY-305 in pancreatitis. Multi-centre double-blind study. *Gendai Iryou*, **12**:261–78 (in Japanese).
46. Ishii K, Takebe T, Hirayama N *et al.* (1984). Clinical evaluation of FOY-305 in chronic pancreatitis. Multi-centre double-blind study. *Gendai Iryou*, **16**:844–54 (in Japanese).
47. Itami Y, Inoue T, Takahashi H *et al.* (1982). Clinical evaluation of elcatonin in the treatment of lumbodorsal pain complicated in osteoporosis. Multi-centre double-blind study. *Igaku no Ayumi*, **120**:1180–95 (in Japanese).
48. Itami Y, Fujita T, Inoue T *et al.* (1982). Clinical efficacy of alfacalcidol (1α-OH-D$_3$) in the treatment of osteoporosis. Comparative study by multi-centre double-blind method. *Igaku no Ayumi*, **123**:958–73 (in Japanese).
49. Shichikawa K, Igarashi M, Sugawara S and Iwasaki Y. (1983). Clinical evaluation of high molecular weight sodium hyaluronate (SPH) on osteoarthritis of the knee. Multi-centre well controlled comparative study. *Jpn J Clin Pharmacol Ther*, **14**:545–58 (in Japanese).
50. Hirohata K, Matsuda T, Watanabe Y *et al.* (1985). Clinical evaluation of CS-600 (loxoprofen sodium) on lumbago. Comparative study with ibprofen by multi-centre double-blind method. *Prog Med*, **5**:1487–505 (in Japanese).
51. Aoki T, Sugawara S, Hoshino T *et al.* (1986). Clinical evaluation of CS-600 (loxoprofen sodium) on osteoarthritis. Comparative study with diclofenac sodium by multi-centre double-blind method. *Igaku no Ayumi*, **136**:983–1001 (in Japanese).
52. Hirasawa Y, Hirashima K, Arakawa M *et al.* (1989). Clinical evaluation of recombinant human erythropoietin (EPOCH) on renal anaemia: A double-blind, three doses comparative study. *Kidney and Dialysis*, **27**:157–77 (in Japanese).
53. Agishi Y, Asanuma Y, Shimizu S *et al.* (1986). Clinical evaluation of lipo PGE, on occupational vibration syndrome using double-blind comparative method. *Rinsho Iyaku*, **2**:1269–89 (in Japanese).
54. Katumura T, Uemichi T, Ohshiro T *et al.* (1986). Clinical evaluation of lipo PGE$_1$ in the treatment of ischemic ulcer of the extremities. A multi-centre double-blind comparison with inositol niacinate. *Junkankika*, **20**:331–50 (in Japanese).
55. Kumagai A, Takahashi S, Shida T *et al.* (1982). Clinical evaluation of HC 20-511 (Ketotifen), a new oral anti-anaphylactic compound, in bronchial asthma. II – Multi-centre double-blind study in comparison with disodium cromoglycate. *Clin Eval*, **10**:737–85 (in Japanese).
56. Kumagai A, Takahashi S, Shida T *et al.* (1980). Clinical evaluation of HC 20-511 (Ketotifen), a new orally anti-anaphylactic compound, in bronchial asthma. I – Multi-centre double-blind study in comparison with placebo. *Clin Eval*, **8**:353–96 (in Japanese).

57. Yasugi T, Goto Y, Yoshida S *et al*. (1988). Clinical evaluation of CS–514, (Pravastatin) on hyperlipidemia. Double-blind study with clinofibrate. *Clin Eval*, **16**:211–49 (in Japanese).
58. Goto Y, Yamamoto A, Matsuzawa Y *et al*. (1988). Clinical evaluation of pravastatin (CS-514) on hyperlipidaemia. Double-blind study with probucol. *Igaku no Ayumi*, **146**:927–55 (in Japanese).
59. Saito Y, Goto Y, Nakaya N *et al*. (1988). Dose-dependent hypolipidaemic effect of an inhibitor of HMG-CoA reductase, pravastatin (CS-514), in hypercholesterolaemic subjects. *Atherosclerosis*, **72**:205–11.
60. Katsumura T, Mishima Y, Kamiya K, Sakaguchi S, Tanabe T, Sakuma A. (1986). Therapeutic effect of ticlopidine, a new inhibitor of platelet aggregation, on chronic arterial occlusive disease. A double blind study with inactive placebo. *Junkankika*, **7**:396–406 (in Japanese).
61. Murakami M, Toyokura Y, Omae T *et al*. (1983). Therapeutic effect of ticlopidine or aspirin on transient ischemic attacks (TIA) – Comparative double blind study for 12 months. *Igaku no Ayumi*, **127**:950–71.
62. *British National Formulary* No 22. (1991). British Medical Association and Royal Pharmaceutical Society of Great Britain.
63. *British National Formulary* No 24. (1992). British Medical Association and Royal Pharmaceutical Society of Great Britain.
64. *Handbook of Medicines*. (1990). A Society for Pharmaceuticals edn. Yakuji Jihou-sya Ltd., Tokyo (in Japanese).
65. Dept. of Social Statistics, Ministry of Health and Welfare. (1992). Summary of medical expenditure in Japan. *Kosei no Shihyo*, **39** (3):32–38. (in Japanese).
66. The Association of the British Pharmaceutical Industries. (1993). *The Health Manager's Guide to the Pharmaceutical Industry*. 1993 edition. ABPI, London.
67. Ohkoshi M, Isigami J, Kamidono S *et al*. (1986). The criteria proposed by the UTI committee in Japan. *Chemotherapy (Tokyo)*, **34**:408–41 (in Japanese).
68. Sakita T, Fukutomi H. (1971). Diagnosis of gastric ulcer. In: Yoshitoshi Y (ed.) *Gastroduodenal Ulcer*, Nankodo, Tokyo, pp. 197–208. (in Japanese).
69. The Official Book Society of Japan edn. (1992). *Guidelines on Clinical Evaluation of Medicines*. Yakuji Nippo-sya Ltd., Tokyo, 1992. (in Japanese).
70. Matsumoto K, Saitoh A, Yokoyama K *et al*. (1977). An assessment method of clinical states in bacterial pneumonia. *Jpn J Clin Pharmacol Ther*, **8**:155–68 (in Japanese).
71. Ohtomo E, Kutsuzawa N, Hasegawa K *et al*. (1982). Clinical evaluation of HOPA (HOPATE) in the treatment of cerebrovascular disorders. – Multi-centre double-blind study in comparison with Ifenprodil tartarate and placebo. *Clin Eval*, **9**:673– 710 (in Japanese).
72. FX-505 project for Phase III study. (1976). Double blind study of FX-505 (Ifenprodil) on cerebrovascular diseases. *Clin Eval*, **4**:419–58 (in Japanese).

73. Kawai K, Kohli Y, Takeda S *et al.* (1978). A multi-clinical double-blind controlled study on the clinical efficacy of proglumide in gastric ulcers. *Clin Eval*, **6**:69–84 (in Japanese).
74. New Drugs Division, Japanese Ministry of Health and Welfare edn. (1990). *Handbook on Good Clinical Practice*. Yakuji Jiho-sya Ltd., Tokyo (in Japanese).
75. New Drugs Division, Japanese Ministry of Health and Welfare. (1992). Guidelines on statistical analyses in clinical trials. *Clin Eval*, **20**:205–219 (in Japanese).
76. New Drugs Division, Japanese Ministry of Health and Welfare. (1992). General guidelines on clinical evaluation of new drugs. *Jpn J Clin Pharmacol Ther*, **23**:609–21 (in Japanese).

6
Ethnic differences in response to pharmaceuticals across Europe

MARISA PAPALUCA

Summary

1. Ethnic variations exist across Europe, and have to be taken into due consideration, but the European regulatory approach enables each Member State to accept all available clinical data for evaluation, including that derived from different European, and even non-European, regions.

2. A project is underway in Europe to compare the clinical safety of some medicinal products evaluated through the Concertation Procedure by assessing data on adverse drug reactions, observed during clinical trials and post-marketing, in each Member State.

3. Preliminary results indicate that the qualitative profile of the detected serious ADRs does not show major differences across the European regions. This suggests that the existing ethnic differences have not had a direct impact on the detection of serious ADRs.

Introduction

Differences in the population response to drugs is a complicated issue to be explored, since these differences relate both to inter-individual variability in pharmacokinetic and pharmacodynamic responses, including a wide range of single subject factors from genetic to psychological and cultural ones, and to external factors. Inter-ethnic differences in metabolic polymorphism may occur, depending on the frequency of certain phenotypes, and to approach this issue in developing a medicinal product at least three different methodologies seem to be promising:

- performing *in vitro* studies on isolated human cells or fractions as experimental metabolic models, which are progressively being validated;
- phenotyping the subject enrolled in the pharmacokinetic studies in order to include both high and low metabolisers;
- including pharmacokinetic parameters from population pharmacokinetic studies in the Phase III trials database.

According to some authors, the inter-racial variation is small compared with that within a single race. However, the possible risks should be balanced with respect to any difference with predictable impact on the clinical efficacy and safety. Variations in both pharmacodynamics and kinetics may give rise to either undertreatment or overdosage in individual patients, which may lead to unexpected interactions as well as adverse reactions.

Ethnic differences in Europe

Europe has several ethnic roots, being a very heterogeneous population with Germanic, Anglo/Saxon, Gaelic, and Latin/Mediterranean groups. In spite of the increasing number of marriages across races, differences among the different ethnic groups have been known for a long time within Europe and it is acknowledged that, for example, glucose-6-phosphate dehydrogenase (G6PDH) deficiency is more common in the Mediterranean area than in the northern part of Europe. Such a genetic polymorphism might influence the pharmacokinetic behaviour of certain drugs which could lead either to differences in clinical responsiveness to those drugs which have a steep plasma concentration/response curve with a narrow therapeutic window, or to a non-difference because of the possibility of titrating the dose according to the level of the desired therapeutic effect. The prevalence of certain diseases might also show large differences, as is the case for hepatitis B which is widespread in Italy, Spain, France and much less common in the UK or Germany, and could lead to different background noise in the baseline values of certain laboratory parameters.

The inter-ethnic differences in response to drugs may also relate to external factors like diet composition (for example, salt and fat intake) or sunlight exposure, which may lead to different dosages and side-effects. But the socio-cultural approach to the diseases themselves can also induce inter-regional differences, with patients keen to seek the doctor's advice and take pills at different stages of their disease because, for example, of the difference in tolerance to pain. The medical tradition also has a great importance, as the scientific language is non-homogeneous, the relationship between the patient and the doctor differs across the different European countries and even because of the different Healthcare Systems and Social Security approaches. In summary, ethnicity, defined as the whole complex of the aforementioned factors, implies the recognition of a sort of specific individual–socio-cultural pattern.

The European Community has been for centuries of history an intrinsically heterogeneous population. However, the improvement of communication and exchanges among the various Member States has already produced harmonisation of some socio-cultural factors. The establishment of common rules and regulatory requirements in the field of pharmaceuticals created the homogeneous background necessary for the harmonisation of the European market. As a consequence of this harmonisation in rules, evaluation of new medicines is carried out in a concerted fashion by all Member States, particularly for those products relating to real innovation. This activity not only led to a better understanding among Member States, but has been driving the medical and social behaviour in a homogeneous fashion across Europe. Considerable effort has also been put into the definition of the Summary of Product Characteristics (SPC), particularly with respect to indications, contraindications, doses and precaution for use.

These regulatory provisions push towards a uniform approach to the use of medicines across Europe. It could be suggested that with the progression of these activities, the relevance of ethnic variations across Europe, *vis a vis* the evaluation of medicine, would not still be an open issue. Differences do exist and have to be taken into due consideration, but it is interesting to note that the European regulatory approach enables each Member State to accept all available clinical data for evaluation, including that derived from trials carried out in different European and even in non-European regions.

In the spirit of the International Conference on Harmonisation (ICH), in order to scientifically quantify the impact of ethnic factors in the acceptance of foreign clinical data, several research projects are ongoing in various parts of the world. One such project is a retrospective analysis being carried out in Europe by the Centre for Medicines Research (CMR) under the auspices of ICH on clinical responsiveness to medicines across the three regions (the USA, Europe, Japan).

European adverse drug reactions study

Another project is ongoing in Europe under the auspices of the European Communities Commission – General Directorate for Scientific Research, concentrating on the impact on clinical safety of some medicinal products evaluated according to the Committee on Proprietary Medicinal Products (CPMP) Concertation Procedure. Pharmaceutical companies were asked to collaborate in this project on a voluntay basis by providing information on the adverse effects observed with their own products, both during the clinical trials (standardised clinical setting in heterogeneous ethnicities) and in the spontaneous ADR reporting systems (non standardised setting in current clinical practice in heterogeneous countries). The cut-off date for the receipt of data was December 1992.

The medicines included in the current review share the same indication, the same dosage and treatment schedule recommendation, and have very similar Product Characteristics (PCs); moreover, the dates of marketing are close in all Member States (1989–1991). The research project is still undergoing the final phase of the assessment of all the data received. Only some of data have been included for the purpose of this review, and the safety profile of the serious ADRs (as defined by the CIOMS I Working Group) and the distribution of the reporting across various Member States have been considered. The drugs were grouped in four classes and for each class only data referring to a single indication have been evaluated.

The spontaneous reporting rate, as expected, varies according to the regulatory and medical framework which is different in different Member States. Nevertheless, as shown in Figures 6.1–3, the qualitative profile of the detected serious ADRs does not show major differences related to the different European regions. In fact, the greater accent on the occurrence of certain types of serious ADRs in the general context of Europe is generally not due to a concentration

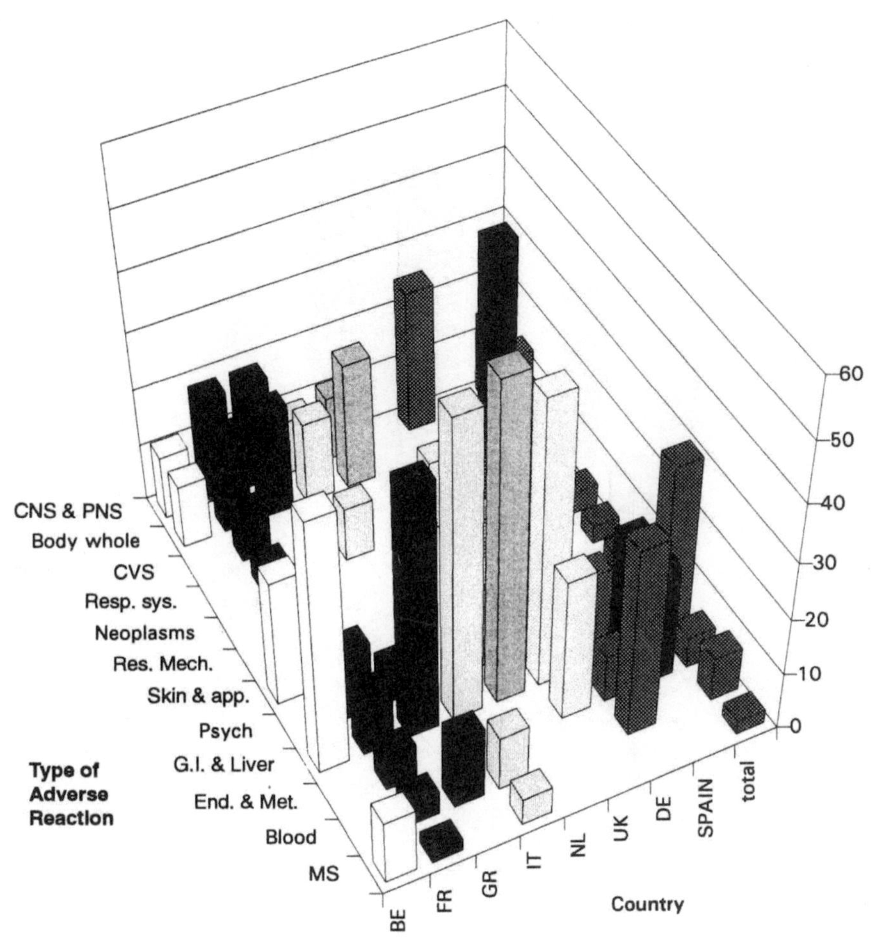

Figure 6.1 Distribution of serious ADRs. Reproduced from Papaluca (1994) with permission

Key:

Type of Adverse Reaction

CNS & PNS: Central and Peripheral Nervous Systems; CVS: Cardiovascular System; Resp. Sys.: Respiratory System; Res. Mech.: Resistance Mechanisms; Skin & App.: Skin and Appendages; Psych: Psychological; G.I. & Liver: Gastrointestinal System and Liver; End. & Met.: Endocrine and Metabolic; MS: Musculoskeletal

Country

BE: Belgium; FR: France; GR: Greece; IT: Italy; NL: Netherlands; UK: United Kingdom; DE: Germany

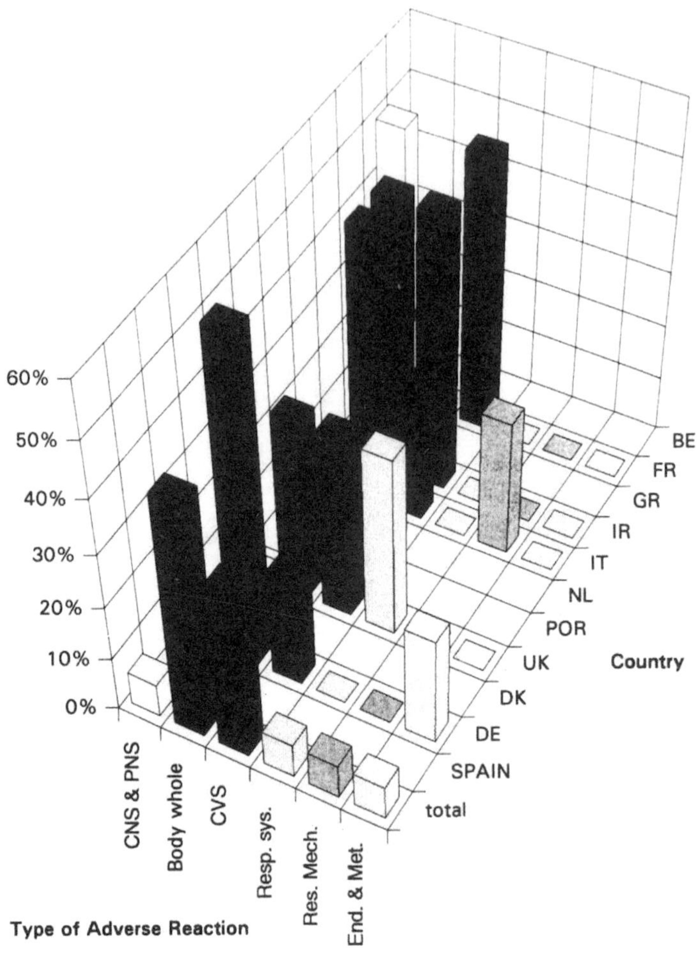

Figure 6.2 Distribution of serious ADRs: Drug B. Reproduced from Papaluca (1994) with permission

Key:
Type of Adverse Reaction
CNS & PNS: Central and Peripheral Nervous Systems; CVS: Cardiovascular System; Resp. Sys.: Respiratory System; Res. Mech.: Resistance Mechanisms; End. & Met.: Endocrine and Metabolic
Country
BE: Belgium; FR: France; GR: Greece; IR: Ireland; NL: Netherlands; POR: Portugal; UK: United Kingdom; DE; Germany

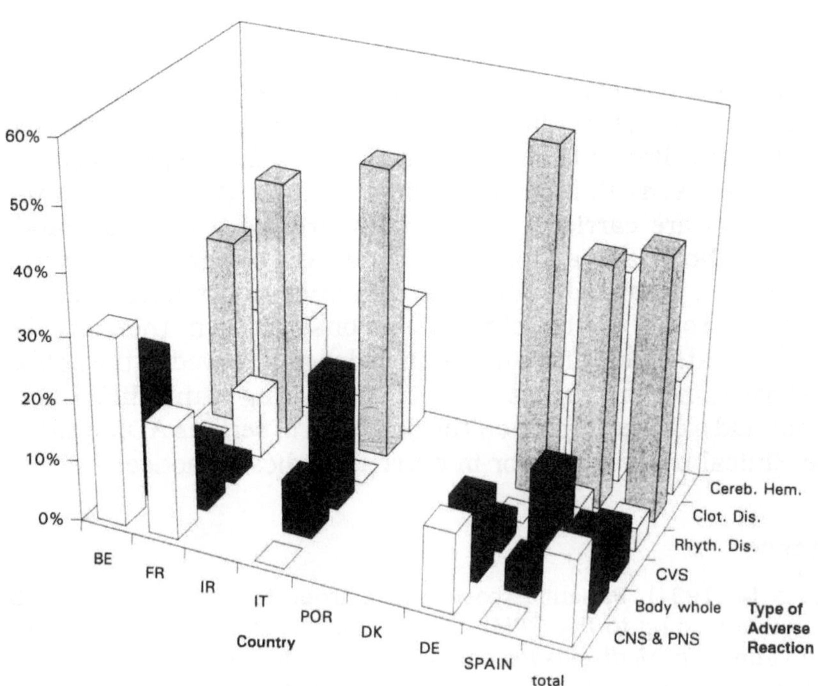

Figure 6.3 Distribution of serious ADRs: Drug C. Reproduced from Papaluca (1994) with permission
Key:
Type of Adverse Reaction
Cereb. Hem.: Cerebral Haemorrhage; Clot. Dis: Clotting Disorder; Ryth. Dis: Rhythm Disorder; CVS: Cardiovascular System; CNS & PNS: Central and Peripheral Nervous Systems
Country
BE: Belgium; FR: France; IR: Ireland; IT: Italy; POR: Portugal; DK: Denmark; DE: Germany

of side-effects in only one Member State or Region, but due to the repetition of the same signal in the different Member States. These findings are of value in the appreciation of the impact of ethnic influences in the perception of safety issues, as the spontaneous reporting systems, particularly in Europe, represent a good model of the non-standardised setting in current clinical practice in heterogeneous countries.

Conclusion

On the basis of this preliminary analysis, no major differences have been observed in the qualitative profile of the serious ADRs reported in multicentre clinical trials conducted across the various Member States. This means that even in different ethnic groups, when the clinical trials are carried out in a standardised way, and standardised methods are adopted to define and report the adverse events, ethnic factors do not seem to induce major differences in the safety profile of the clinical response. It can therefore be concluded that, at least for this group of drugs reviewed in the actual regulatory framework across Europe, the existing ethnic differences have not had a direct impact on the detection of serious ADRs, either in the clinical trials setting or in current medical practice.

Reference

Papaluca M (1994). Patient exposure in Europe to medicinal products evaluated according to the CPMP Concertation Procedures. In: Fracchia GN (ed.) *European Medicines Research: Perspectives in Pharmacotoxicology and Pharmacovigilance*. EC-IOS Press. (in press 1994).

7
Medical practice differences between Europe, the United States and Japan

JOHN HENDERSON

Summary

1. The assessment of the relationship between benefit and risk in respect of drug use is different between Japan, Europe and the United States. In Japan, safety is given a greater weighting relative to efficacy than in the other two geographic regions.

2. The assessment of the benefits of medicines also differs in Japan. Clinical trial design more closely equates with clinical practice and there is a greater emphasis on the subjective judgement of the individual physician, compared with the situation in Europe and the United States. The introduction of statistical guidelines, as well as those for GCP and the more recent guidelines on clinical trials, clearly demonstrates the desire to harmonise the standards of drug development in Japan with those of the West.

3. In the United States, proof of efficacy requires a minimum of two separate well conducted clinical studies showing statistically significant superiority of the investigational drug for the indication sought over the comparative agent, whether placebo or active substance. Therapy is more aggressively pursued with higher levels of risk being acceptable than would be true in Japan.

4. Europe lies between the extremes of Japan and the United States with the practice of medicine influenced significantly by the culture of the country concerned. Diagnoses made in one country sometimes have no exact parallel in other European countries and there are marked differences in prescribing patterns across Europe.

5. Differences in medical practice currently prevent acceptance of Japanese clinical data in the West and vice versa. However, change is beginning to occur, albeit slowly.

Introduction

Although modern day medicine in both Japan and the United States of America can trace its origins back to Europe, the practice of medicine in these three areas differs greatly. Indeed, there are marked differences in medical practice within Europe itself. How does this come about? Professor Anthony Clare wrote an editorial in the *British Medical Journal* in 1989 under the general heading of "National Variations in Medical Practice" (Clare, 1989). The specific title was "Culture Influences Medicine More Than Science Does". This article reviewed a book written by Lynn Payer in which she espouses the theme that the practice of medicine in the United States, West Germany, France and Britain is influenced more by national characteristics, cultures and philosophies than by scientific consideration (Payer, 1988). Although the book was criticised, having had personal experience of observing medical practice in Europe, in Japan and the United States, I would argue that the basic thesis put forward by Lynn Payer is true and that it applies to Japan as well as to the countries mentioned in her review. To attempt to do justice to this complex philosophical topic and to describe how it impacts on clinical drug development and dosage levels is no easy task.

Japan

Having lived and worked in Japan for just over two years, I have little more than a superficial understanding of the complex culture that characterises Japan, which is very different to the West. The following are some personal observations on some aspects that seem to impact the practice of medicine and to affect the process of clinical drug development in Japan.

The assessment, in respect of drug use, of the relationship between benefit and risk is different between Japan, Europe and the United States. In Japan safety is given a greater weighting relative to efficacy than in the other two geographic areas. This directly reflects Japanese culture and its requirements in respect of inter-individual relationships and obligations. Given that the concept of benefit/risk assessment underlies the whole drug development and approval process, it should not be surprising that the greater emphasis on lack of risk relative to efficacy should often lead in Japan to a determination of recommended dosage levels lower than in the West. However, the situation is made more complex because of the hierarchical nature of Japanese society. The medical profession has a very high standing. Indeed, in this respect, Japanese society is very like many of the individual European societies of earlier this century. Such a hierarchy seriously inhibits free communication between doctor and patient. Informed consent to participation in a clinical trial has only very recently been demanded by the introduction by the Ministry of Health and Welfare of Good Clinical Practice (GCP) requirements, issued first in draft form in 1985 and implemented on October 1st, 1990.

Communication between doctor and patient is still limited. In normal clinical practice, it is not uncommon for a doctor to see upwards of 100 patients during a morning or afternoon clinic. The incidence of side-effects reported in the application for marketing approval for a drug, used at the same dosage level in Japan, the United States and Europe, was reported by Homma at the First International Conference on Harmonisation in Brussels (Homma, 1992). Because of differences in the way these data were collected, particularly in respect of attribution to study drug, it is hard to draw definitive conclusions. However, the overall incidence of reported side-effects is lower in Japan. This is evidenced also by comparison of data sheets from Japan and the West for other drugs, and by the data presented by Naito (1994). In the past this comparison has frequently been confounded by differences in the recommended dosage. It can be concluded that communication between doctor and patient in Japan does not result in the identification of as many adverse events as in the West, although this conclusion does not apply to *serious* adverse events. The overall lower incidence of reported adverse events, despite the greater emphasis in Japan on safety, is more typical of normal everyday practice of medicine.

The benefit side of the equation is also evaluated differently in Japan as discussed by Hirokawa and Dollery (1994). There is a greater emphasis on the subjective judgement of the individual physician, and of the Assessment Committee of senior investigators who collectively review and evaluate the data for individual patients prior to data analysis. In double blind trials this review is conducted prior to the breaking of the double blind randomisation code by the independent controller for that study. A simple example of this process of evaluation may be offered by the Guideline, issued by the Ministry of Health and Welfare, for "Clinical Evaluation of Antihypertensive Drugs" (Anon, 1986). This is one of many guidelines issued by the Ministry describing in great detail how to develop a drug in a given therapeutic category. The description of these as "guidelines" is misleading to the Westerner: they are rules and departure from them has to have an excellent and sustainable justification. It is relatively unusual to include a placebo control group in Phase II or Phase III studies. In the latter, a single study per major indication, it is required that when available there be an active comparative agent of appropriate mode of action and author-ised indication to compare to the drug under study. In Phase II, an active comparator is also more likely to be used than placebo, although placebo is not proscribed. This tendency to avoid placebo, in marked contrast to the United States, reflects the desire of the individual physician to ensure that his or her patient receives, even during a clinical trial, appropriate therapy for the underlying con-dition. Thus, in the criteria set for the objective evaluation of antihypertensive therapy in Japan, there is only passing reference to placebo response.

Clinical assessment

Various methods may be used for assessment:
- Fall in blood pressure relative to baseline:
  The mean of two baseline and of the final two visit measure-ments are compared.
- Classification of the quantified fall in blood pressure, relative to baseline as put into one of seven categories ranging from "marked fall" to "marked rise":
  A marked fall is one of at least 30 mmHg for systolic pressure and for diastolic pressure of at least 15 mmHg etc.
- Assessment based on a fall in blood pressure of at least 20/10 mmHg, relative to baseline, plus the absolute blood pressure values obtained at the end of treatment:
  This is viewed as an important assessment in a flexible dose study. This particular assessment is not used, however, in the elderly or in patients with complications because the achievement of a blood pressure within the normal range in such subjects may be hazardous.
- Evaluation of the overall antihypertensive effect throughout the treatment period:
  The hypotensive effect is rated as excellent when the blood pressure curve shows a slow fall and produces few fluctua-tions in the treatment period.

Adapted from Anon (1986)

In addition to these assessments, the first three of which are objective, the investigator will make an overall evaluation of antihy-pertensive effect, grading the response into one of five categories taking into consideration:

"Comparison of the hypotensive effect, degree of difficulty in controlling the blood pressure, blood pressure curve and values of the blood pressure at the end of treatment".

The Assessment Committee of senior investigators will also make their own evaluation of the antihypertensive effects based on the individual patient assessments as well as the mean data. So despite an objective endpoint, lowering of blood pressure, the primary efficacy endpoint is *subjective*.

As in all therapeutic categories there is also an overall assessment of safety, that is side-effects and laboratory data. While the assessment of side-effects is subjective, that for laboratory data is not. There are clearly established criteria, for example, in the guidelines describing antibiotic development, that define quantitatively various levels of abnormality. Compared to the West, relatively minor changes are regarded as clinically relevant. Further, these assessments of efficacy and of safety are combined into an evaluation of the overall usefulness of the new drug. The Guideline describes in detail how the overall utility should be classified into one of six categories using these assessments of safety and of efficacy. The sixth category, "use prohibited", is used for all patients in whom treatment was stopped early because of adverse findings or events. As I have suggested above, the system described bears an obvious relationship to how the individual physician manages, in normal clinical practice, an individual patient. The overall results for the two treatments, the investigational drug and the comparative agent, are compared with the emphasis on overall usefulness.

Statistical evaluation

Until relatively recently, even a single, statistically significant advantage for the investigational drug was sufficient to allow approval and to obtain a small price premium over the competition. Such a marginal advantage is no longer sufficient. Statistical guidelines have now been introduced by the Ministry of Health and Welfare (MHW, 1992). Given the relative lack of placebo controlled studies in Japan, the Ministry of Health and Welfare has tackled the difficult problem of determining what constitutes a demonstration of efficacy for an investigational drug when compared to an existing active therapy. The Guideline makes clear that the lack of statistical difference does not prove the equivalence of the two treatments. Two methods for verifying clinical equivalence are described. Both require that there is a predetermination of the level of the clinically acceptable difference, Δ, between the investigational drug and the positive control drug. This, it is suggested, will vary with disease and drug effect, but a rough guideline of 10% is offered. The two statistical methods are:

(1) The investigational and positive control drugs are judged clinically equal to each other if the confidence interval for efficacy differences between the two drugs (90% confidence interval) does not cover the range narrower than Δ (the predetermined clinically allowable difference).

(2) One tailed hypothetical testing (significance level: 5%) is done for the null hypothesis that "the effect of the investigational drug is inferior to that of the positive control drug by more than Δ". The two drugs are judged clinically equal to each other if the hypothesis is rejected.

These verification methods are intended to assure equivalence by proving that the effect of the investigational drug is not inferior to that of the positive control drug by more than Δ. However, the Ministry of Health and Welfare recognises the deficiencies of this method and in the introduction to the Guidelines requests input to allow a better method to be devised.

The introduction of these statistical guidelines, as well as those for GCP and the more recent still Guidelines on Clinical Trials, clearly demonstrates the desire to harmonise the standards of drug development in Japan with those of the West. However, these Guidelines also serve to demonstrate some of the problems that remain. While the clinical trial guideline proposes a minimum of eight patients per centre, this is not achievable without a radical change in the way drugs are developed. Even senior members of the medical profession have criticised this as an impossible number to achieve and the pharmaceutical industry also sees difficulties with this proposal. The present system of conducting multicenter studies in large numbers of discrete centres, with the majority perhaps recruiting less than six patients, prevents an analysis of variance with site as a variable. This is the traditional method of drug development and in large measure reflects patient availability. Further, as clinical studies are prohibited during the NDA approval process, the current design of multicenter studies is the only way a pharmaceutical company can obtain a reasonable number of doctors with experience of the new drug at the time of launch.

United States

While in Japan the conduct of clinical trials closely follows how the individual physician might treat his patient in normal practice, in the United States a different situation applies. There the study of a new drug requires the most rigorous application of the current, most appropriate and valid methodology to the assessment of the new drug. Proof of efficacy requires that there be, as a minimum, two separate well conducted clinical studies showing statistically significant superiority for the investigational drug for the indication sought over the comparative agent, whether placebo or active comparator. The determination of the optimum dose range requires complex dose response studies in which the study drug is often prescribed in a way that is different from how it will be used subsequently in clinical practice. There are several examples of drugs approved at a given dose range in the USA but for which much lower dosages have become the norm in the marketplace. I am not aware of this phenomenon in Japan.

Why are there such marked differences? American society tends to be confrontational and aggressive, adjectives that could not be applied to Japan where collective harmony is critically important. These societal characteristics may require the Food and Drug Administration to publicly defend any of its decisions. Food and Drug Administration officials must ensure that they can fully justify their decisions under such public scrutiny. This means a lengthy and detailed review of all the data submitted in a New Drug Application (NDA) to ensure that all analyses are appropriate, that data are correct and accurate, and developed in accordance with Federal Regulations. This aggressive approach by American society is also reflected in the way doctors use drugs. Therapy is aggressively pursued with higher levels of risk being acceptable than would be true in Japan, to allow achievement of therapeutic goals. Further, society demands that there has to be full and informed consent by the patient. American culture forces enormous investments in drug development by industry and by the Federal Government; over 2000 employees at the Food and Drug Administration are involved in new drug development and approval processes. This contrasts with Japan where the entire New Drugs Division of the Ministry of Health and Welfare has only 21 staff dealing with NCEs. However, they have an enviable record of productivity in terms of numbers and speed of NDA approvals.

Europe

Europe lies, in many respects, between the extremes of Japan and the United States. Yet the practice of medicine is impacted significantly by the culture of the country concerned. Europe does not have a homogeneous culture. Marked cultural variations in Europe are reflected in marked differences in clinical practice. There are diagnoses made in one country which have no exact parallel in other

European countries. There are marked differences in prescribing patterns across Europe. The most frequently used drug in Italy is a digoxin preparation, in Germany a nasal decongestant and in the UK an anti-asthmatic. Not only are there differences in the types of drugs prescribed, but there are also differences in preferences for routes of administration. In the past such differences have made it difficult to construct a clinical development programme for Europe without significant country specific components. But the situation is changing. This is not because medical practice *per se* is changing significantly but because of harmonisation activities within the European Economic Community and the European Free Trade Area. For many years before international harmonisation became fashionable, the Committee for Proprietary Medicinal Products (CPMP) within the EC and, initially separately, the Nordic countries and Finland had been working to develop guidelines for the clinical and preclinical development of the drugs in many different therapeutic categories. In consequence of these activities, it is now possible to have a single registration dossier of common content that should meet the requirements of all regulatory authorities throughout Europe. This does not mean that there are no individual country-specific requirements, nor a common standard of review. This latter is readily evidenced by the enormous range of questions asked at national level by individual regulatory authorities, although a common database had been filed (Harvey *et al.*, 1993). In turn this offers some insight into the problems of the current non-binding process for new drug approvals using CPMP. How this will change with the establishment of the European Medicines Evaluation Agency and the implementation of new directives in 1995 remains to be seen. However, the differences in national and medical culture in Europe are beginning to have less impact than previously on the clinical drug development process. Could this same trend extend to encompass the United States and Japan? Eventually we shall see more clinical harmonisation but more is only a relative term. The cultures of the United States and Japan, in particular, are so far apart that any process of harmonisation, at least at a clinical level, will be slow.

Ethnic differences

There is still a strongly held view that there are important ethnic differences between Japanese and Westerners that impact on both pharmacokinetics and pharmacodynamics. However, the problem is that because a difference is expected to be present, the presentation of data to the contrary is met with some scepticism. If it were possible to show unequivocally, at least for certain chemical series or even therapeutic classes, that kinetic and dynamic differences do not exist, will this allow for harmonisation? The primary issue is not ethnic difference or lack thereof, but the differences in medical culture and practice. It is quite clear that for the foreseeable future the practice of medicine in Japan will not allow a clinical drug development process compatible with that in the West. This has nothing to do with the Market Oriented Sector Selective (MOSS) Agreements which require that Phase I ADME, Phase II dose range finding and Phase III comparative studies be conducted in Japan in Japanese patients. Rather it is because of the medical culture, of the way medicine is practised.

Good clinical practice requirements in Japan

The most obvious difference in these guidelines relative to those that are legally binding within the EC and those that are contained within the Federal Register in the United States, is in the relative responsibilities of the sponsor, i.e. the pharmaceutical company, and of the investigator. In Japan, a senior physician will take responsibility, at the request of the pharmaceutical company, as chief investigator either for a programme or, more frequently, a study. The chief investigator, who will be both scientifically and politically influential in the therapeutic area under study, has the primary responsibility for protocol design, for overseeing the conduct of the study in accordance with GCP requirements and for furnishing a report of the study. However, while the sponsor company will provide the resource to monitor the study, it is the chief investigator who has overall responsibility, not the sponsor company. The chief investigator thus makes a major investment of time and reputation in the drug in question. Further, he will not support departure from the processes described in a therapeutic guideline, where this exists, unless there is a very sound and justifiable reason for so doing. This can be a source of difficulty as for example with the development of an anti-arrhythmic, the guidelines for which were issued many years before Cardiac Arrhythmia Suppression Trials (CAST) and reflect the thinking prevalent prior to that study. But perhaps more than anything else, the stumbling block to harmonisation of clinical programmes is the tradition that in clinical studies, evaluations should equate closely to normal everyday medical practice. Clinical trial design and endpoints reflect this practice of medicine rather than rigorous scientific experiments measuring objective endpoints. Even before consideration is given to differences in assessment of benefit/risk, it is evident that the methods used are likely to lead to differences in the labelled dose in Japan relative to the West. However, change is taking place. The ICH process is leading towards harmonisation of GCP between Japan, the United States and Europe. Further, even without introducing significant changes in the practice of medicine, it should be possible to make progress. In the West, for antihypertensive drugs we collect baseline and end of treatment data. An approach which allows analysis of these objective data, whether of Japanese or Western origin, should be possible. Use of these analyses as the primary efficacy endpoints would require Koseisho, the Ministry of Health and Welfare, to amend its guidelines and persuade the medical profession to accept this change. Such changes will take place, but the process will be slow.

References

Anon (1986). Guideline for clinical evaluation of antihypertensive drugs. In: *Guidelines for Clinical Evaluation of New Drugs*. Yakugyo Jiho Co. Ltd, Tokyo.

Clare, A (1989). National variations in medical practice. *Br Med J*, **298**:1334.

Hirokawa K and Dollery CT (1994). The top 50 drugs in the UK and Japan: why are they so different? In: Walker SR, Lumley CE and McAuslane JAN (eds) *The Relevance of Ethnic Factors in the Clinical Evaluation of Medicines*. Kluwer Academic Publishers, Lancaster, pp. 63–88.

Harvey C, Lumley CE and Walker SR (1993). A comparison of the review of a cohort of NCEs by four national regulatory authorities. *J Pharm Med*, **3**:65-75.

Homma M (1992). Requirements for assessment of clinical safety regulatory perspectives. In: D'Arcy PF and Harron DWG (eds) *Proceedings of The First International Conference on Harmonisation, Brussels, 1991*. The Queen's University of Belfast, pp. 390–399.

MHW (1992). *Guidelines on Statistical Analysis of Clinical Trials*. Ministry of Health and Welfare, Japan.

Naito C (1994). Evaluation methods for clinical trials of drugs in Japan which may affect ethnic differences. In: Walker SR, Lumley CE and McAuslane JAN (eds) *The Relevance of Ethnic Factors in the Clinical Evaluation of Medicines*. Kluwer Academic Publishers, Lancaster, pp. 49–62.

Payer L (1988). *Medicine and Culture*. Henry Holt & Co., New York.

8
A survey of current practices in the US regarding minorities and gender: the pharmaceutical perspective

LIONEL D EDWARDS

Summary

1. The number of clinical trials required for a new drug application has increased over the past few years due to the addition of special studies including those involving pharmacokinetic data, clinical pharmacology, drug interactions and special clinical population studies such as geriatric patients and those with renal impairment.

2. Increasing concern over the possible absence of data in women and minority groups led to a survey of current industry practice on this topic among PMA member companies. Thirty-three companies out of forty-six operating in the United States (71%) responded to the survey. Ninety-four percent of the responding companies always collect data on gender and 79% record the race of patients or volunteers.

3. Seventy-nine percent of the respondents claimed that the FDA had prevented the inclusion of fertile women while 67% reported such a request by an institutional review board. Forty-four percent however recorded requests by the FDA and 30% by international agencies to include more women in NDA submissions.

4. The findings from this and other surveys confirm that differences between gender and race in the handling of drugs is only rarely found.

Introduction

The number of clinical trials required for a New Drug Application (NDA) or to support additional indications has continued to increase. By 1989, an average of over 60 studies for each NDA were being filed and this was reflected in data from an increased number of patients submitted (3567 on average, Boston Consulting Group, 1993) (Figures 8.1 and 8.2).

Phase III studies have become smaller in number but larger in size. Thus, the overall increase in the total number of studies is due to the addition of special studies including those involving pharmacokinetic data, clinical pharmacology, drug interactions and special clinical population studies such as geriatric patients and those with renal impairment, etc. Now, with requests for adequate representation of women in the NDA database and also minority representation, neither the number of studies nor patient numbers are likely to decrease (FDA, 1988).

The cost of bringing a new drug to the market for the average American company has been reported as \$230 million (Di Masi *et al.*, 1991) . A survey by the Centre for Medicines Research of 13 major trade associations revealed that the total R&D expenditure by the international pharmaceutical industry in 1993 was estimated to be in excess of \$26 billion (Walker personal communication). As about 50 new chemical entities are approved each year and this has remained constant over the past 20 years, this means the cost is about \$500 million for each new medicine although only about 80% of all R&D expenditure is for new drug discovery and development. These escalating costs result in expensive medicines and new requirements will add to this, which is why international efforts to reduce duplication are so important.

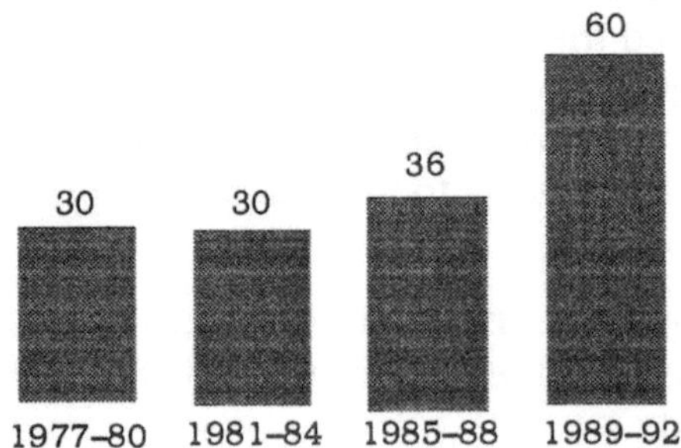

Figure 8.1 Clinical trials per NDA. Adapted from BCG (1993)

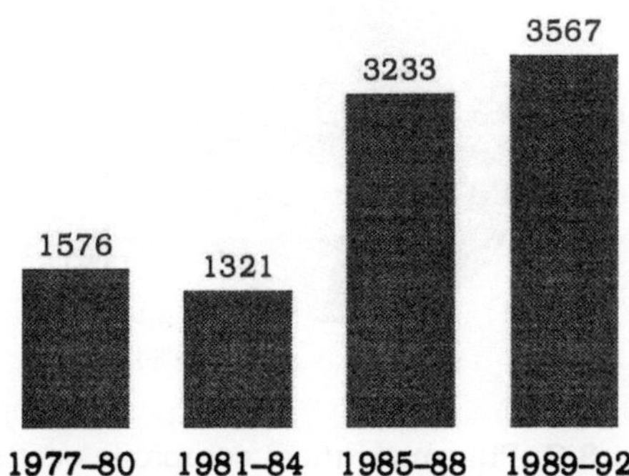

Figure 8.2 Clinical trial patients per NDA.
Adapted from BCG (1993)

In 1989, when I was appointed Chairman of the PMA Special Population Group, I detected an increasing concern over the possible absence of data in women and minority groups. The perceived problems arose out of their conspicuous absence in longitudinal epidemiology or treatment outcome studies rather than an overwhelming evidence of differences in efficacy and safety for gender and race in short-term drug studies. The issue was partly political and revolved around "natural justice", "rights" and methodology issues. A survey of the current industry practice of gender and minority inclusion was undertaken among PMA companies. The questionnaires were returned anonymously with each participating company sending back a postcard separately to indicate they had provided a response.

Results

Thirty-three companies out of 46 operating in the USA (71%) and representing the largest American and international companies responded to the survey. The results are expressed in terms of the percentage of responding companies. Ninety-four percent of responders always collected data on gender. Seventy-nine percent always recorded the race of patients or volunteers (Figure 8.3), but only 30% frequently recorded data on menses. Seventy-seven percent recorded US racial groups, i.e.: Black, Caucasian, Hispanic, Asian, and/or Oriental in the majority of studies. Native American Indian/Eskimo were only recorded by 48% but this could reflect the small incidence in the US population (0.8%) (Figure 8.4).

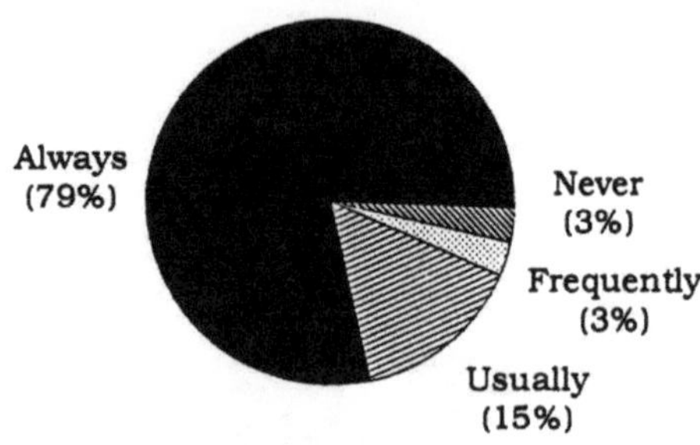

Figure 8.3 Pharmaceutical companies collecting data on race

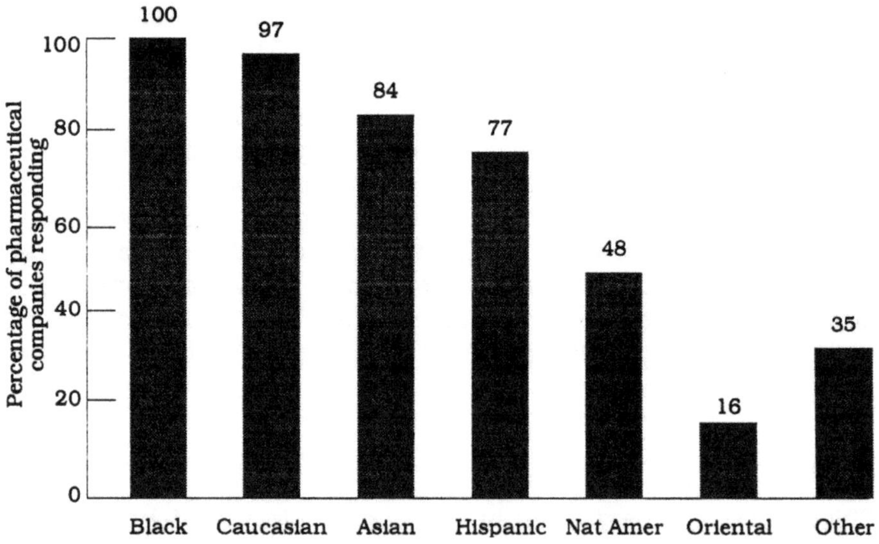

Figure 8.4 Pharmaceutical companies collecting data on racial populations

The prevention of studies in fertile women resulted in significant differences. Seventy-nine percent claimed that the FDA had prevented the inclusion of fertile women, 67% reported such a request by a board or Institutional Review Board (IRB), and 35% by international agencies (Figure 8.5). Generally this was in Phase I and II clinical studies. Forty-four percent of respondents, however, also recorded requests by the FDA and 30% by international agencies to

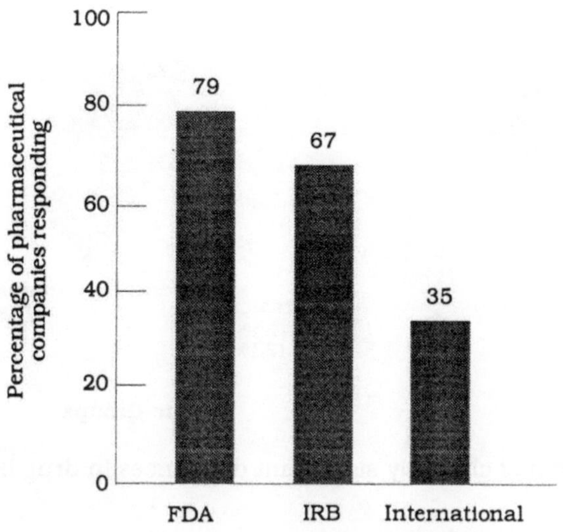

Figure 8.5 Exclusion of fertile women (by agency)

Figure 8.5 Exclusion of fertile women (by agency)

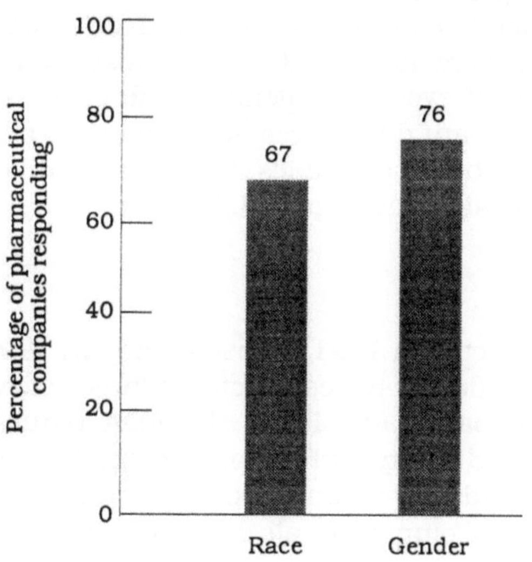

Figure 8.6 Pharmaceutical companies showing effort
to include special populations

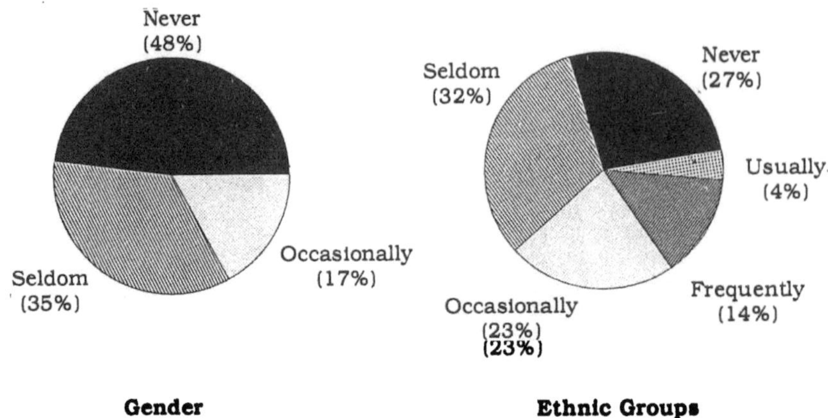

Figure 8.7 Detection of clinically significant differences in drug handling

recruit more women into NDA submissions. Both the FDA and international agencies were reported by 30% of companies to occasionally request the inclusion of racial groups. Sixty-six percent of companies tried to recruit more women and 67% tried to increase racial representation in their studies (Figure 8.6). The success of these efforts was not recorded although there had been adverse reports by the FDA and General Accounting Office in their surveys. The survey included questions with respect to how often significant gender and race differences in response to a drug's clinical effect (efficacy and safety) were found. Although most companies responded that seldom, if ever, were gender differences seen, 17% occasionally saw significant differences between males and females in drug handling and these companies indicated antihypertensive drugs as the commonest agent (Figure 8.7).

Discussion

This survey was conducted in 1991. Subsequently in 1992, the US General Accounting Office (GAO) conducted a larger survey which included smaller companies. In 1988, the FDA requested data analysis for efficacy and safety with respect to gender and race be included in the NDA and they recently examined the data on drugs submitted since 1988. Common to all three reports is the finding that differences between gender and race in handling drugs are only rarely found. The GAO indicated that this could be because it is rarely sought but the bulk of evidence emerging today refutes their view. The incidence of significant differences for both gender and race is likely to be less than 5%.

There remain many unanswered questions, the most important is whether it is worth the extra time, money, and potential delay to examine every drug for racial and gender differences. Politically, it would appear expedient to do so and new FDA guidelines are being issued and a Congressional Bill submitted (FDA, 1993; Schroeder *et al.*, 1993). Two-hundred and fifty patients have been suggested in the GAO report (GAO, 1992) as constituting a reasonable sample. This of course would vary with respect to the effects to be detected and the toxicity of the drug which may be unknown early in development. Which racial groups should be included or excluded? Hispanic is an ethnic group made up of many racial origins. Already some North American/Eskimo centres have declined to be involved especially in "me-too" drug studies. The Black population is also very suspicious of the predominately "white" research community which can influence recruitment and patient response. It has also been suggested that population pharmacokinetic (PK) screening in Phase II or III may suffice. However, given the inevitably small numbers in some groups, the chance of spurious results will increase. The final question is whether these results, either negative or positive, found in populations of considerable racial and ethnic intermarriage, are applicable to less mixed groups such as the Japanese or French.

Conclusion

With the new FDA guidelines just issued, the industry is expected to include adequate numbers of patients with respect to both gender and major racial groups although it is uncertain as to how small the sub-groups can be. The value of such data is also questionable. Currently, the US industry recruits irrespective of race or gender, but in the future it will have to be more proactive in this respect. Menses data, where applicable, should also be collected and oral contraceptive interaction studies undertaken. My conservative estimate of the extra costs of recruitment, additional studies, PK work, analysis and reports would be between $3 and $5 million. In addition, a potential delay of about two months might also be expected. Now that the FDA is to encourage the participation of potentially fertile women in clinical drug studies, the gateway for increased potential liability has also been opened. The ultimate cost of all these measures will be reflected in the increased cost to the patient, insurers, government agencies, and, ultimately, the tax-payer.

References

Boston Consulting Group (BCG) Report (1993). The Changing Environment for US Pharmaceuticals. The Role of the Pharmaceutical Companies in a Systems Approach to Healthcare. Sponsored by Pfizer Inc. Available on request (USA).

Di Masi J, Hansen R, Grabowski H and Lasagna L (1991). The cost of innovation in the pharmaceutical industry new drug R&D cost estimates. *J Hlth Econon*, **10**:107–142.

Food and Drug Administration (FDA) Department of Health and Human Services Public Health Service (1988). Guideline for the format and content of the clinical and statistical sections of new drug applications. *Federal Register*, Volume, 53, October 1988.

Food and Drug Administration (FDA) (1993). Guideline for the study and evaluation of gender differences in the clinical evaluation of drugs. *Federal Register*, Volume 58, July 1993.

General Accounting Office (GAO) (1992). Women's health: FDA need to ensure more study of gender differences in prescription drug testing. GAO, October 1992, Washington DC.

Schroeder P, Snowe O and Mikuisici B (1993). Pharmaceutical Testing Fairness Act (HR 2695) Section M Congressional Proposed Bill. Women's Equity Act of 1993.

9
Current approaches to global drug development from a European perspective

JOHN PATTERSON

Summary

1. In view of the current costs of new drug development, for a company to be successful it must have a strategic plan for the global development of its new chemical entities.

2. Global development can be defined as an attempt to reach all major markets as rapidly as possible in a cost effective and efficient manner. For some companies this will include the United States, Japan, Germany, France, Italy, UK and Canada which represents approximately 85% of the developed pharmaceuticals world.

3. Successful global drug development should result in a single data sheet/package insert with one set of utility statements for the product. Unfortunately, differences in medical practice including differences in diagnosis, treatment and clinical research methodology in various countries can swamp all the attempts to achieve a global programme. Ultimately, meaningful clinical harmonisation between Japan and the Western World, although seemingly remote at the present time, would have a significant impact on the global development of new medicines.

Introduction

In this paper the problems of global development of new chemical entities are discussed with respect to ethnic variation, although at times it presents a superficial view of some aspects of the development process. There is little data which shows that patients from different ethnic backgrounds respond to medicines in any clinically meaningful different ways. There are differences, but these do not appear to be clinically significant.

In addressing the development process, the first thing to be aware of is that a European based pharmaceutical company, such as Zeneca based in the UK, has a different set of problems to many other pharmaceutical companies which are situated in much bigger markets such as the United States or Japan. If the home market comprises less than 10% of the world market, even a company that has a large share of it cannot recover the R&D costs there alone so it is necessary to enter the bigger markets as soon as possible to ensure the medicines that are being developed are viable. With a small base there is a strategic imperative to be international and to globalise development. Given the current cost of drug development, it does not matter how big the home market is, companies still have to be international.

Secondly, although the UK is part of Europe, even the European market itself is not necessarily a large enough entity nor is it even a single entity. While the concertation process has been established and changes are being enacted to standardise registration within Europe, there really is still, from a medical perspective, no single European market. There are many "ethnic" differences, amongst them diversity of medical culture, language barriers and pricing issues. Furthermore, with the costs of medical care generally becoming unacceptable to health providers, many changes are being introduced such as "need" clauses and black lists that start to work against even the best, standardised, harmonised, concertation process. These forces act to prevent companies getting their products into the market places of Europe quickly and effectively.

Some regulators and physicians are nationalistic and they still want to see evidence that the medicine that they are registering has been used in people of their own race and cultural background. The pharmaceutical industry has to recognise and accept this at the same time as we are trying to use resources efficiently and prevent unnecessary duplication.

Definitions

The term "global development" is widely used. It will be defined in two ways. One is that "it is an attempt to reach all major markets as rapidly as possible (because time is important in relation to patents) in a cost effective and efficient manner". This means trying to do work that is internationally acceptable rather than just for one country, with a data package that does not simply obtain registration but enables successful marketing. The importance of the latter statement is that it means addressing pricing issues and comparisons with important standard agents in an attempt to define a place in medical practice.

The second definition is equally important. Although many outside the industry may think we are financially well endowed, resources are finite within even the biggest company. Decisions have to be made on how to use resources for which there are always excess demands. As a result, many potentially good medicines never get to the market place. Global development may also be defined as "using international resources and expertise to allow the company to reach a (clinical) decision point rapidly and effectively with the minimum human exposure that allows the decision to be made safely and effectively". This stopping process is just as important in global development because the lost opportunity costs of pursuing something into Phase III that ought to have been stopped in Phase II or the human costs of continuing something that has an unacceptable profile are just as important to a company in terms of its success in a highly competitive environment.

The first definition of global development leads to two possibilities. Firstly, many people think in terms of a single worldwide clinical submission, in other words a single harmonised package that is sent to every country in the world at the same moment in time. That is the "holy grail" of development and it certainly has the attractions of time saving and efficiency of resource utilisation but is often unrealistic. Secondly, a more practical solution is a global evaluation programme which is harmonised. This is still attractive because it provides access to patient populations, it spreads regulatory risks (for example, if a regulatory authority stops a clinical programme, it allows you to be continuing your work elsewhere), it allows you to submit trials applications in some countries that give approvals earlier or do not need approval, whilst waiting for others that do. So there are good reasons to operate internationally that are not simply about producing a single international package. My definition of "global" is to work towards approval in the USA, Japan,

Germany, France, Italy, the UK, and Canada, which represent approximately 85% of the developed pharmaceuticals world. If we can introduce a product rapidly into those markets, then, assuming it meets its profile, it is likely to repay its development costs. While we focus on registration in only six or seven countries, we undertake clinical development work in considerably more countries because many of them have extremely good medicine, high standards and provide data that is acceptable in the bigger countries.

Geographical spread

Zeneca is undertaking global regulatory work in sixteen sovereign States scattered through five Continents. The work is deliberately spread over those States for a number of reasons. It may be the medical excellence of these countries, or that they are an important market, for example, France, Germany and North America. It may be that there are regulatory requirements (often unwritten) that mean a submission will not be accepted as a package without some patients from that country. Some countries such as Australia are seasonally out of phase with the Northern Hemisphere for diseases such as asthma or hay fever, thus extending the annual recruitment period. Recently our regulatory clinical trials have been extended into Hungary and Czechoslovakia and they have produced impressive work and data. These countries have both survived an internal FDA style GCP inspection and come out with flying colours. They have not had a real FDA inspection yet, but sometimes getting through the company review is more difficult than getting through the FDA one. These countries have another attraction in that they are not saturated with products under development, which means easier access to patients and shorter recruitment times, a key issue in large international trial programmes. Finally, Zeneca works in Japan in parallel with the rest of the world but this work does not contribute to the global development unless adverse events occur.

Planning

Successful global development should result in a single data sheet/package insert with one set of utility statements for the product. These result from a well controlled set of studies which are harmonised into a set of overviews. The nightmare of the past was where, for over a decade or more, compounds were being developed independently around the world resulting in different data sheets, different indications and different dose regimes.

Companies spend a great deal of time before starting the first study working through the planning, organisation and design of an international integrated programme. We consult with leading experts in the world and talk to the key health authorities. From there we develop a plan with the intention of producing a single international regulatory package, and this is under our control.

Some of the problems that are faced in trying to execute a core international clinical trial plan, with particular reference to ethnic differences in medical practice, will now be described. Two other important impediments are regulatory issues from the outside and internal corporate and logistic issues.

Regulatory issues

Regulatory controls clearly impact on our activities. For example, the control processes for clinical trials can be divided into permissive and restrictive systems. For the same study, some countries simply will not give approval to start whereas, in other countries, approval does not have to be sought and studies can start straight away. A classic permissive example would be Phase I studies in healthy volunteers in the UK which are not covered by the UK Medicines Act and do not therefore require regulatory approval. Sweden has a restrictive system and approval can take many months. That means that not all centres in a programme can start on the same day. In addition, there are different toxicological requirements for different phases of clinical development throughout the world, and in the past countries like Italy have been unable to take part in Phase I and early Phase II trial programmes because of relatively restrictive requirements compared to the rest of Europe. The Italians are changing their law at the moment and moving into line with the rest of Europe. This also illustrates that a country may change its laws overnight, totally changing the accessibility of patients in either direction.

"Take-over bids" by some of the major health authorities can also be a problem. When a trial programme has been designed and discussed with many experts and is then presented to the regulators, there is somebody there who knows better than you exactly how your drug should be developed and tells you how to do it. The company can be faced with a dilemma when there are specific, sometimes conflicting, requests from individual health authorities. These requirements have to be built in or ignored at your peril. They can also impact on the integrity of the programme.

When the licence application is submitted, there are differences in both content and presentation requirements. Regulatory requirements for dose ranging studies vary as do the definitions of adequate and well controlled studies and the need for local work and comparators. There are a series of international registration requirements which, although becoming more harmonious, still represent significant differences to the licence applicant.

Comparing and contrasting the UK and the US regulatory activities in Phases II and III provides a view of the difficulties that a company faces in running a single international regulatory programme. The UK has a permissive study initiation process (although it is not as simple as Germany, where the data is simply submitted and the study started) compared with the Investigational New Drug (IND) system which is more restrictive. An added complication is that if clinical trials supplies for the global programme are sourced from the USA, exporting the material can be difficult, so one country's restrictions can affect the rest of the world. There is, however, a downside to the permissive programmes in that there may be no dialogue with the health authority or only summary documentation is reviewed and, as a result, the company does not acquire any feedback on potential issues or problems that may be coming at the time of the licence application. In contrast, an authority like the FDA will have gone through all the documentation and given a real insight into the perceived problems prior to approval. The danger is, of course, that somebody different may review the package two years later and form a different opinion. Nevertheless, an opinion is obtained, whereas in the UK and the other permissive systems, this is not available.

Company issues

It is sometimes more difficult to get international harmonisation within the company than it is with the regulatory authorities. Companies, like any large group of people, have power struggles and internal politics. There is nationalism (we now call it cultural diversity), there is national pride and there are organisational issues, all of which interact with attempts to run a coordinated international programme. Even such a seemingly simple thing as the ability to dispense material from clinical trials dispensaries throughout the world can represent a major logistical issue which sometimes slows the programme down or puts different parts of the programme out of phase.

Medical practice

I believe that the impact of differences in medical practice swamps all of the effects of other issues on a global programme. This is dealt with under the sub-headings of diagnosis, treatment, research methodology and healthcare systems.

Diagnosis

Diseases may be diagnosed more frequently in some countries than others due to a greater prevalence, for example, the incidence of stomach cancer in Japan. There are also different diagnoses which simply are not recognised in certain countries. In Germany, a diagnosis of hyperkinetic heart syndrome is not uncommon, but a Danish or a Swedish physician probably would not be able to define this. The French complain of feeling "liverish" and in the UK "headaches" appear to be a national euphemism for when people feel slightly unwell. Those differences in national disease patterns and diagnosis clearly have an effect on an international programme. They can cause serious problems in certain therapeutic areas, for example, schizophrenia. While the diagnostic criteria are being harmonised through the Diagnostic and Statistical Manual of Mental Disorders, 3rd Edition, Revised (DSM3R), there are other diagnostic instruments which can be used in different ways to obtain the diagnosis. Having recently sat with 150 US psychiatrists and watched them trying to resolve inter-rater variability on the Brief Psychiatric Rating Scale (BPRS) and Scale for the Assessment of Negative Symptoms (SANS) rating scales from a series of video tapes of US patients, the variation of interpretation was enormous, even within the US medical culture. Again, while diagnosis of hypertension has now become international, differences between use of Korotkoff 4 & 5 have had to be ruled out. In contrast, for diabetic neuropathy, there are no standard diagnostic or measurement criteria at all.

There are ethnic differences in the availability and use of diagnostic tests. For example, in breast cancer, oestrogen receptor measurement is taken as a standard measure in the USA, but it is hardly available outside the United States. For many tests, hospitals have their own laboratories and standards, clinicians also have their own laboratories and different standards. It is possible to get around variability by using central laboratories but it becomes a very expensive and huge logistic exercise moving blood samples all around the United States or Europe. Nevertheless, companies do it as a means of standardising the process and this is also one way of compensating for variability in and increasing the precision of a geographically diverse programme.

Infectious disease represents a unique problem because there are different patterns of pathogens internationally, different resistance patterns of these even between hospital and the community within a country as well as between countries. We see transatlantic differences in the definition of septicaemia and bacteraemia. These are minor but important differences if a trial programme is being run and information is to be pooled. Unless those differences can be reconciled and harmonised, a heterogeneous collection of information will result, which is very hard to describe in a licence application and makes writing the claim structure a formidable challenge.

Treatment

Having achieved international diagnostic standards, even greater hurdles lie ahead in the way that different medical cultures approach the use of the test drug and the concomitant medical therapy or the comparator agents. One example relates to the use of haloperidol in schizophrenia. The usual regimen in the US is less than 15 mg per day while France indicates that unless 15–30 mg per day is given, patients are clearly under dosed and that they could neither participate in a study at the US dose nor use it for regulatory approval. There are major issues in blinding a comparator and the existence of different formulations. A recent interesting experience involves a progestational agent. In order to undertake a double blind comparison with our agent, we bought the comparator, reformulated it into a double blind formulation and then undertook the bioequivalence study against the standard drug. The competitor company had a standard medicine in Europe and another in the USA, supposedly using the same formulation with only a colouring agent difference. We found that their two versions were in fact bioinequivalent and although we showed that our reformulated comparator was bioequivalent with one of the two, it was not equivalent to the other, so two years' work was wasted and finally an open label study had to be conducted.

Differences in medical practice in areas like asthma and heart failure turn transatlantic programmes into a mine field. The pattern of use of low dose inhaled steroids early in treatment in Europe in contrast to the US makes recruiting steroid naive patients into a European trial programme almost impossible. In schizophrenia, again it is necessary to run a placebo comparison in the acute treatment of schizophrenia in the United States whereas in Europe that is considered unethical and it is necessary to use a low dose of the test substance as a "placebo arm", which it clearly is not. Again it prevents a company from bringing the programmes together in a standard fashion. Problems can occur in therapeutic areas like hypertension in the use of step therapy or switch therapy and, of course, single or multiple drug regimens. Some countries will use many drugs at low doses in an attempt to keep down the side-effects (Japan and Germany are two of those countries) while others disapprove of fixed combinations, such as UK and Scandinavia where higher doses of monotherapy are more commonly employed.

An interesting international difference in the whole philosophical approach to treatment exists in the cancer area. There is no doubt that west of the Atlantic an aggressive approach in cancer is certainly seen as the key, stemming from the log kill hypothesis for cytotoxic agents. When oncologists start applying that philosophy to a cytostatic endocrine therapy for cancer it starts to become less meaningful. Nevertheless, that does happen. The European approach is usually less aggressive and the view of a UK oncologist of the 1970's on tumour therapy was that "the tumour should really shrink faster than the patient" for the treatment to be of any value. Quite a different view to his US colleagues, who found his approach unacceptable.

Research methodology

At one time I had the pleasure of running a study in Japan comparing an oral anti-oestrogen with a parenteral androgen entitled "a double blind study", without even the second "sham" injection. The study was perfectly acceptable as the double blind study for regulatory purposes, but to non-Japanese eyes, it looked a rather strange thing to be doing.

Even when a definition of the disease and the treatment has been made, response criteria can vary significantly. For example, for prostate cancer, the European Organisation (EORTC) has its own definition of partial and complete response, different to the East Coast Oncology Group, even though they are using the same measures. How can a transatlantic trial programme be written up only once in such circumstances? We have, on some occasions, simply defined (prospectively) a company hybrid response criterion which has been accepted by health authorities.

The philosophy of good clinical practice (GCP) is now widely spread throughout the world, only differing in some of the detail. International studies can be run to GCP standards in most areas of the world and it is not an impediment to international activities. It is one area where recently there has been significant harmonisation and the guidelines for Europe, the FDA and WHO are very similar.

Adverse event reporting is an important issue for the pharmaceutical industry. We have recently run a trial programme of a Japanese antibiotic in Europe and the USA, with about 4500 patients recruited into the European and US programme and a similar number recruited in Japan. The Japanese programme yielded 47 significant events, the European and US programme revealed 10 times that number. The pattern was the same in both data sets but the threshold for reporting and the relationship that the doctor has with his patient and with his health authority is clearly different. Certainly, when marketed products are examined, quite significant differences in the reporting rates are seen throughout the world. Japan, again, has one of the lower report rates per head of population in spite of their high usage of medicines. The UK has one of the higher ones. On the whole, we have not experienced any adverse events that were unique to a particular ethnic group although they may have been reported earlier and more often in one culture than another. This issue of acceptance of risk/benefit is important and this is what leads to the desire for low doses in some countries, particularly Japan and Germany. It is an attempt to do no harm and creates diametrically opposite pressures to those generated by other countries that demand maximal efficacy with a tendency to push the dose upwards. This is particularly true when small numbers of very large, expensive trials are to be undertaken. There is a great desire in this situation to run with the highest possible dose to avoid "missing" the potential utility of the test substance.

Healthcare systems

Healthcare systems have a major effect in perturbing international coordinated programmes. They mandate things such as local pricing studies. The comparator and dose that is used for pricing studies vary with locality and can form a second barrier to registration which can also be an invisible trade barrier. Medical care systems impact on what work is done and where. With an office practice system rather than the polyclinic system, there are much smaller numbers of patients in any centre which can lead to statistical problems. Office based doctors tend to have rather less sophisticated equipment, although not in every country. The availability of ancillary research staff varies with the system. Some physicians run a professional trials organisation. That has disadvantages as often the same resistant patients go through every trial but it has the advantage that they are professional about what they do. They also have staff who understand GCP and about the keeping of records and filling in the record forms.

Who owns the patient's medical records in a country? Is it the patient, is it the government, or is it the doctor? Who has a right to inspect those patient records? Whether it is a representative of the company or somebody from a health authority requiring access alters the rules, and that is taking some sorting out in certain countries in relation to the source data verification requirements of GCP.

Finally, the method of payment for healthcare has a major effect on some of our activities, and an illustration of this is given for an intravenous anaesthetic. With an agent that gives rapid recovery, day case anaesthesia was seen in some countries as a tremendous advantage for the patients, hospitals and the health system by eliminating an expensive overnight stay. In other systems it was a disaster because the hospital was paid for every night that the patient spent in bed and if the patient was sent home at 5 o'clock in the afternoon, the hospital did not get paid and they did not like it. When this anaesthetic was first developed, Japan was not interested. The underlying rationale was that Japanese anaesthetists are paid at two different levels for a minor and a major anaesthetic. The difference was considerable and depended on whether an endotracheal tube is passed and the patient ventilated. The Japanese anaesthetist was resistant to the idea of using a new agent administered with a light intravenous technique which did not always require intubation compared with the standard inhalation agents. As a result, the programme is running some eight years later in Japan than the rest of the world.

Finally, the role of an expert is quite different throughout the world and one has to understand how different cultures perceive their role in the regulatory process. In caricature, the USA regards the expert as a "hired gun" and when you take an expert to the FDA, they have no doubt he is representing you, even though he presents a balanced independent view. It is quite often a question of their experts against your experts in an adversarial process.

In Japan the Clinical Trial Committee (the CTC) is run by an expert professor who actually runs the programme and decides if the product works, so he is very important and has a major influence on the registration process. In Europe the expert is somebody of substance who reviews the database and then writes an expertise which is supposed to be his own critical assessment of the data and claims. His view is, in the main, respected. These are three quite different approaches to the expert. If you take a European expert to the FDA you really have to make him understand his role before he goes.

Development in Japan

Meaningful harmonisation in the clinical area in Japan seems remote at the moment. All of the programmes that Zeneca will be running to the end of this century will be as self-standing Japanese programmes that will include any existing non-Japanese data at the time of submission but it will be seen as supportive data only. If the NDA and the UK licence have been granted, that is helpful but the Japanese programmes will be self-standing. The Japanese work is run one to two years behind the rest of the world for several reasons. One is to save resources and reduce the failure rate. The 'n' value for Phase I studies in Japan is almost always less than 10 and so the chances of being able to achieve meaningful Phase I and early Phase II data with a high enough statistical power to be self-standing is low. In our experience, non-Japanese data is needed to get into the correct dose range before starting in Japan. The preclinical work for Japan has generally been slower although we are now managing to bring it back in line with the West.

Individual Japanese studies are also getting bigger, but overall the regulatory programmes are still relatively small, comprising 500 patients or less for all the phases. There are problems of concomitant therapy, global rating scales and dose. There are several examples of dose differences where ethnic factors are cited but are really irrelevant. An example of this situation is the decapeptide which is a luteinising hormone releasing hormone (LHRH) analogue and binds to the gonadotrophin releasing hormone (GnRH) receptor on the pituitary gland. If enough of this relatively non-toxic decapeptide is given, it down regulates the receptor and switches off luteinising hormone (LH) and follicle stimulating hormone (FSH) and the sex hormones. In prostate cancer a dose well above the top of the dose response curve is administered to ensure down regulation as there are no obvious dose related side-effects. It was suggested by colleagues in Japan that the dose should be reduced

Table 9.1 Japanese clinical developments (NCEs)

Year of NDA	Clinical development	Approval time
76	6 y 1 m	2 y 3 m
80	4 y 7 m	1 y 4 m
80	4 y 1 m	2 y 10 m
89	5 y 2 m	2 y 4 m
89	4 y 1 m	1 y 8 m
92	4 y 1 m	
—	5 y 2 m	
—	5 y 5 m	
—	4 y 8 m	

to the threshold dose. However, it was difficult to persuade them that the dose needed to be well above the threshold for inhibition with a monthly depot as any loss of control by day 28 would result in transient tumour stimulation in the next cycle. A half strength depot which fulfils Japanese needs for benign gynaecology where breakthrough is not such an important problem is now being developed. There is another agent being developed in the West at 150 mg while colleagues in Japan feel that 80 mg is absolutely imperative. The argument given is that the blood levels at 80 mg are not different to the Western 100 mg blood levels, which is true, but when there is an 'n' of 4 in Japanese Phase I, the type 2 error risk is really quite significant. A pragmatic approach is taken to these problems to get the programmes moving and there is no evidence that the patients in Japan have suffered as a result of the minor differences that one sees with the way the products are used, but it makes it impossible to harmonise the work.

Products brought through Japanese development by Zeneca are shown in Table 9.1. Clinical development times have come down slightly to about four to five years in the Japanese system. These data are only for New Chemical Entities (NCEs) and do not include new indications. The approval times are reasonable.

Zeneca's approach to global development

The objective is to get products through to market safely and quickly. A template has been set within Zeneca for the whole of development, including clinical, with milestones and standards irrespective of the product, and this template is used for all developments. There are international teams and management processes and a production line approach to the work. The activity is seen as a standard process into which there is intellectual input that is product specific but which is amenable to improvement through production techniques.

For trial design and content, the FDA is considered as our key regulatory authority. The USA represents 30 to 40% of Zeneca's world market so their needs must be met as a minimum. A clinical development organisation is distributed to achieve "global" activity, although the budgets are centralised to control these activities.

A single package is filed for Europe, first line markets and the USA. There are 17 first line markets that accept the regulatory package without prior approval in the UK. It is ensured that all clinical trials wherever run in the world are reported only once, which means a standard approach to writing up clinical trials is needed, as well as a standard international publishing process. In fact, we only analyse and report regulatory trials in the UK or the USA, wherever they are performed. There are standard interpretations of summary data and the package insert is based on what we call an essential information document so that the proposed claims and warnings are absolutely standardised worldwide. Again, once the company interacts with health authorities, some changes are mandated and the data sheets then differ from country to country.

Although a single global development leading to one regulatory package is attempted, what often results is a rolling, customer-focused series of filings especially for multi-indication products such as antibiotics and cancer drugs. The reason is that it is necessary to be realistic and do what is achievable rather than setting out to do the optimum and getting nowhere. Unfortunately, repeatedly assembling and reporting data packages is expensive and time consuming and in one case the regulatory package was rewritten three times in 18 months.

One problem within Zeneca lies in getting the international project management activities right and many companies find this such a problem that they do not attempt to bring Europe and the US together. However, the US is so important for Zeneca that an international project physician (IPP) is appointed for every project supported by an international biometrician. The person may be located in the USA or Europe and the IPP heads a therapeutic team with biometrics and data handling which brings the project together functionally. Organisationally they are brought together too, with a monthly line management meeting and a host of planning and

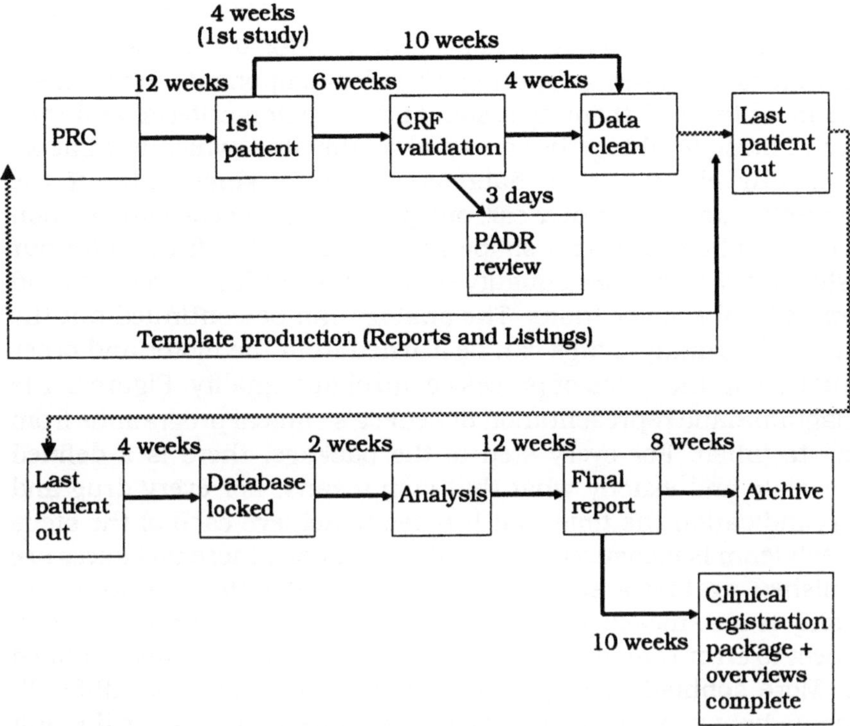

Figure 9.1 Medical function target timings

coordination activities. Japan sits somewhere outside this process with separate reporting relationships.

An idea of the kind of workload that results from this approach is indicated by the fact that in 1993 studies in 3000 clinical trial centres were planned or undertaken. There is a major US focus with 1000 of those centres in the US and 1850 in Europe. This wide geographic spread leads to a major logistic exercise with over 900 people in the medical function of the company spending about 25% of its R&D budget on its medical activities this year.

It is important to regularly review the processes and to seek efficiency. The clinical trials process has been run using car manufacturing as a model. What have clinical trials got to do with, for example, the Ford Motor Company? Well when they build a motor car (our regulatory package) they have a series of suppliers who provide gear boxes, engines and wheels and we have a series of clinical trialists who supply patients and clinical data. They never rely on one source otherwise if there is a strike, they stop making motor cars. We too have to rely on multiple centres and distribute our sourcing. We have to set specifications for our trials through the protocol, they design specifications for components. We both set tolerances (we call them inclusion and exclusion criteria) and they have to bring it all together on an assembly line, which is what we do on our clinical trials database. Their product rolls off the production line as a motor car, our product is a licence application that has to be the correct shape and size and specification for our customers. We both need quality control, QA, multiple products and to meet local specifications. The analogy can be continued but the point is that many things can be learned from the motor and other industries in the areas of process control and quality. Figure 9.1 is a diagrammatic representation of Zeneca's clinical programme from start to finish. For every step of the package, there is a defined time-scale and exactly what that step means. For every drug and every indication the time that it takes to achieve each of the steps in each team is measured. On a quarterly basis, these measures are published against a series of target timings within the function. Quality is also measured, which is more difficult, but possible with respect to error rate in record forms, fields unfilled, headers unfilled etc. More sophisticated quality measures are even more difficult, such as how many protocol amendments were made after the first protocol, or how many times the protocol was changed to increase the recruitment rate? Those things give an indication of the thinking that went into the work and, of course, the final quality measure is whether the product was approved and was found to be safe and effective in clinical practice.

Conclusion

While a global evaluation programme is achievable, some therapeutic areas are easier than others and there are many pit falls. In an ideal world, all the studies would start simultaneously with standard protocols and ethics committees would meet every week. The Institutional Review Board (IRB) requirements would be met, trial materials would be delivered to everybody simultaneously with infinite shelf life, trialists would have enough eligible patients, the data would come in clean, the players would not change the rules throughout a five-year programme and a single package would be then submitted worldwide. As this is unlikely to happen at least in the next few years, a pragmatic approach to individual customer's needs within a global evaluation process is most likely to succeed.

10
Current approaches to global drug development from a Japanese perspective

BRIAN A GENNERY

Summary

1. For many years, the focus of Japanese pharmaceutical companies was entirely on the home market. However, recent changes in the environment in Japan have started to make Japanese companies look to overseas markets as the area for future growth. This has resulted in a change in their approach to global drug development.

2. There are a number of options available for developing new markets for any company and these include licensing out and cross-licensing, the establishment of a liaison/representative office, setting up a development centre with R&D facilities, joint ventures, affiliated operations and mergers and acquisitions. Traditionally, companies have used the first and second of these options but others are now being actively pursued.

3. For foreign owned companies, understanding the regulatory process, the culture and medical practice in Japan is essential to efficient drug development in that country. For Japanese companies, the major problem is that until now local data could not be used as part of the clinical efficacy package in North America or Europe as the clinical research process differs substantially to the rest of the world and there are differences in good clinical practice. Thus, there are major obstacles for a Japanese company moving into the area of global drug development.

Introduction

For many years the focus of Japanese pharmaceutical companies was entirely on the home market. The approach to global development was for the inventor to develop the product for the Japanese market and at some point during the development process to seek a licensee to develop and market the product in almost all other territories. If a single licensee was not involved, a number of different licensees might be used for different territories.

Recent changes in the environment in Japan have started to make Japanese companies look to overseas markets as an area for future growth. This means that their approach to global development is beginning to change.

The Japanese environment

Japan is the second largest pharmaceutical market in the world after the United States. It has traditionally been a high priced market and the development process was relatively simple with the Ministry of Health and Welfare making known its requirements very clearly, in terms of the types of studies to be done and the way the data was to be presented.

One of the reasons for the large size of the Japanese market and its rapid growth, is the dramatic change in the demographic pattern which can be seen, particularly in the very elderly age group over the age of seventy-five. Figures 10.1 and 10.2 present the over sixty-five population as a percent of the total for the years 1950 projected through to 2020, and the same data for the over seventy-fives. As can be seen, Japan has had the most dramatic growth in these groups and as these groups are the biggest consumers of healthcare resources, the Japanese market has grown faster than most others. In addition to being big consumers of healthcare resources, they are also the population that suffer the most from chronic disease thereby insuring good revenues for companies that discover products that are suitable for treating such diseases.

The second reason that the home market was so attractive to Japanese companies was that the pricing process and structure meant that a new chemical entity almost automatically had a price premium over its most recently introduced competitor. As doctors are both the dispensers as well as the prescribers of drugs and much of their income is derived from their sale of drugs, it is not surprising that there was a rapid switch to new high price products as they became available.

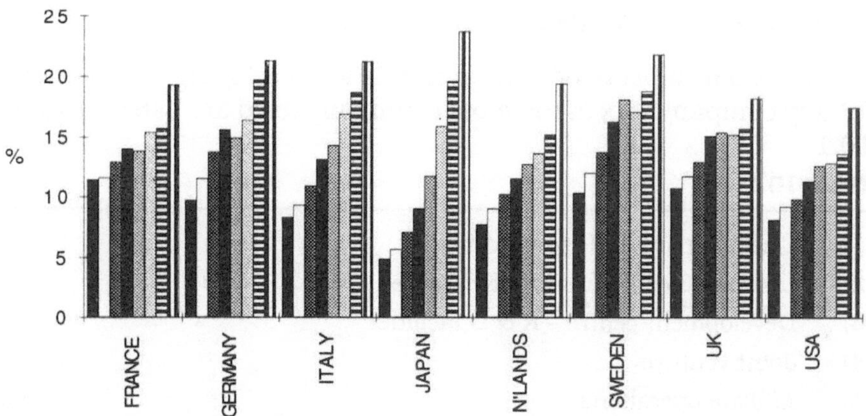

Figure 10.1 Over 65s as a percentage of the population 1950–2020 (columns are decades). Adapted from Chew (1992)

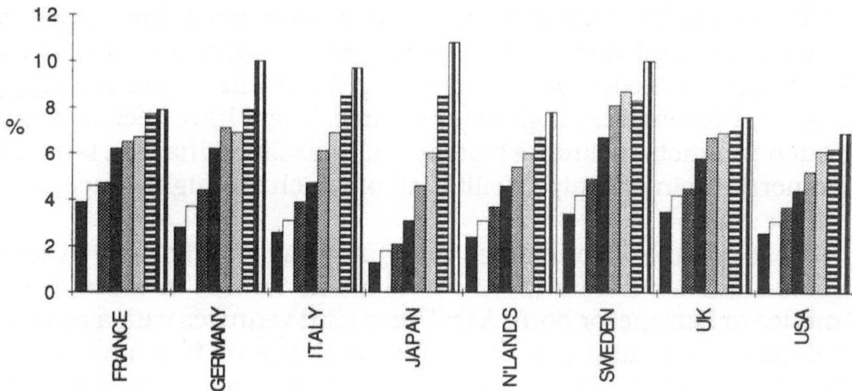

Figure 10.2 Over 75s as a percentage of the population 1950–2020 (columns are decades). Adapted from Chew (1992)

The key change which has happened in Japan over the last few years is that this automatic price premium is no longer available and for products to attract a higher price it is necessary to demonstrate some kind of real benefit.

Thus, the motivation now exists for Japanese pharmaceutical companies to start developing products on a global basis.

Options available for developing new markets

There are a number of options available for developing new markets for any company. Six of the most commonly used are listed in Table 10.1.

Table 10.1

---

(1) Licensing out and cross licensing

(2) Liaison office/Representative office

(3) Development centre – R & D facilities

(4) Joint venture

(5) Affiliate operations

(6) Mergers and acquisitions

Traditionally, Japanese companies have used the option of licensing out and this has been a successful approach for many of them with some compounds achieving the status of market leader, or at least having very high sales volume. There have been a variety of such products including bleomycin, cefazolin, diltiazem, famotidine, norfloxacin and piperacillin, all of which are highly successful in their class.

Most Japanese companies now have liaison offices or at least representative offices and/or development centres in either North America or Europe, or both. A few have joint ventures with a number of different international companies and one or two have set up affiliate operations. In Europe, at least, these have tended to be by companies that have products coming into niche markets where a relatively small sales force and marketing team will be adequate to sustain the products. There are two or three examples of mergers or acquisitions having taken place, but as yet no company has launched a product through an acquired company. So how successful this type of approach is going to be is not clear. Probably, an acquisition is the only way to acquire a retail size sales force for products which are suitable for general practice prescribing. To build up an operation capable of promoting and supporting a number of retail products as a stand alone affiliate operating company would take many years and the investment required would probably be far too high. Add to this the fact that in Europe this would have to be multiplied many times over and it becomes very clear that few, if any, companies would have the will or the resources to make such an undertaking.

Issues and opportunities

The issues for Japanese companies trying to move into the area of global development are exactly the same as any other company, namely:

Understanding the regulatory process

Whilst this is a common problem for all, it is particularly perplexing for people looking at it from Japan at the moment. Whilst the FDA is very rigorous and demanding, at least it is only one agency. In the European Community it is possible to get misled into believing that everyone is working under a single system, where in fact there are nuances of differences between the Member States and then one has to wrestle with the problems of the Multistate and the Concertation Procedures. Finally, this whole process is in a period of transition to the new systems with nobody quite knowing how they will work out.

Understanding the medical culture

Here we are dealing with differences in approaches to clinical trials with the greater acceptance of the use of placebo, a different approach to dosing, which is driven more by obtaining maximum efficacy than by the avoidance of side-effects and the fact that the investigators in Europe and North America now accept the idea of company staff monitoring and auditing on a regular basis.

Understanding local medical practice

Whilst there are many examples of new products being introduced in North America and Europe, where there has been rapid and wide acceptance of their use in the medical community, such explosive take up is the exception rather than the rule. Most practitioners in the Anglo Saxon countries at least, are relatively conservative in their approach to the use of new products, and newness in itself is not reason enough to even start using a product. A company has to normally demonstrate that it has a particular value over what is already used by the practitioners. This is in contrast to Japan where new products tend to get taken up relatively quickly at the expense of old products, but in return they have a relatively short product life cycle.

Understanding the problems of pricing and reimbursement

This could be the subject for a whole paper by itself but in essence, from a Japanese perspective one is looking at an enormously complex and varied series of both written and unwritten rules for pricing a product within the European Community countries. Notwithstanding the problems of pricing, the issue is then of ensuring the product is going to be reimbursed by the State. If the latter is not achieved, clearly the product is going to have only limited success. As the procedures and processes for overcoming these two hurdles are often complex and subtle it is not surprising that executives in Japanese companies are somewhat puzzled by them.

The question then arises as to whether Japanese companies are in a better or worse position to tackle the problem of global development in the light of these issues. The first problem is that until now local, i.e. Japanese, clinical data has not been able to be used as part of the clinical efficacy package in North America or Europe. This is for many reasons. The first is that the Japanese clinical research process differs substantially with the principal investigator being very much the driver of the whole process and this individual also is totally responsible for the selection of co-investigators. They take a very important role in the development of the protocol and the strategic plan. They are also responsible for carrying out the analyses and drawing the conclusions.

The second area of difference is in Good Clinical Practice where there are four major areas of difference. These are:

(1) *Ethics Committees (IRBs)* – Japanese Ethics Committees do not operate in a way that would be recognised as satisfactory, either by the US IND Regulations or European GCP guidelines.

(2) *Consent Process in Japan* – This is very much less structured than either in Europe or North America and is almost never written.

(3) *Source Data Verification* – This is very difficult indeed and in some ways meaningless as the principal investigator is the prime driver of the whole process.

(4) *Centre and Patients* – Each centre contributes only a few patients (usually between one and five) to the protocol and thus would not stand up to the statistical requirements expected in GCP standard studies in the Western world.

Thus, for global development purposes there needs to be a fundamental change in the way Japanese clinical trials are to be carried out if they are to be part of a global package at least for the purpose of efficacy.

The clinical process in Japan has meant that the costs of clinical research are relatively low with company medical departments being very small and the virtual absence of medical advisors, field clinical research associates or many of the other functions which are now normal in any Western company. This is reflected in the research and development expenditure of Japanese companies as a percent of sales. The R&D spend of all Japanese companies in the year 1980 as a percent of sales was 5.5%, in 1985: 7% and in 1988 it was 6.9%. If one took only the companies who are members of the Japanese Pharmaceutical Manufacturers Association this number would be somewhat higher, but still in the region of only about 10 or 11%. This can be contrasted with the 1991/92 R&D spend of the ten leading companies in Europe (Table 10.2), where the average is clearly in the upper teens with Roche reaching 23% of sales. Thus, for Japanese companies to make a big impact in the West they are going to have to spend much more on the R&D function particularly the clinical investigation areas of development.

Table 10.2

Company 1991/92	R & D spend ($mill)	Sales ($mill)	R & D as % of sales
Glaxo	1052.70	7247.00	14.50
Roche	953.30	4119.90	23.10
BMS	845.00	5908.00	14.30
Hoechst	785.8(1)	6263.90	12.50
Bayer	688.8(2)	5306.40	13.00
Ciba-Geigy	677.8(3)	4052.30	16.70
Sandoz	675.00	4440.70	15.20
SB	654.60	4370.10	15.00
J & J	569.00	3795.00	15.00
B-Ingelheim	462.80	2534.50	18.30

(1)   relates to health division, including cosmetics
(2)   relates to healthcare division, including diagnostics
(3)   relates to prescription pharmaceuticals

Reproduced from Thorpe (1992) with permission of the publishers of *Scrip World Pharmaceutical News*.

The main part of this investment is going to be in the need to set up local R&D facilities. Whilst this might be relatively straightforward in the US (if somewhat expensive), when it comes to Europe there are a number of other challenges that need to be faced. Although with the completion of the single European Act it would appear that Europe is now acting in total harmony when it comes to pharmaceutical matters, in reality this is not true, particularly when it comes to the question of pricing and reimbursement. These functions are very much left to individual governments to determine and as a government's decision may well be taken on the basis of input from local leader opinion and the results of local clinical trials, it is still necessary to look at Europe as a somewhat fragmented continent.

The one major advantage that Japanese companies have at the moment is that they do not have significant or affiliate groups in position. This means that they can start with a clean agenda and not be trying to impose a clinical development process on top of an organisation that has for many years been acting as a series of independent units. The areas of learning that are necessary for a Japanese company to start operating in the multinational environment, particularly of Europe, are language, culture, business process, investment needs and medical R&D spend.

Conclusions

Thus, it can be seen that there are formidable obstacles to a Japanese company moving into the area of global development. However, it is important to remember a number of features about Japanese companies, the first of which is that they think very strategically. Therefore, they are willing to make shorter medium-term sacrifices in order to achieve their long-term goal. Secondly, they always approach new situations very cautiously. They are very thorough in their analysis of the situation and the requirements needed to be successful in it. They almost always try and put themselves in a 'win win' situation. Thus, with their natural caution but willingness to work strategically, it is very likely that they will be as successful as anyone in global drug development.

References

Chew R (1992). *Compendium of Health Statistics*, 8th Edition, 1992, OHE, London.

Thorpe T (1992). Merck and Glaxo vie for top spot. *Scrip Review*, 1992, pp. 16–17.

11
Summary of Session I

TREVOR JONES

This paper summarises the key points made in Session I and highlights some of the issues that require further discussion. The principal point is that, with few notable but perhaps clinically important exceptions, it is probable that intra-ethnic variation is a greater issue than inter-ethnic differences.

Types of genetic polymorphism

There are varying types of genetic polymorphism, as described by Professor Breimer. Firstly, it could be regarded as an inherent unalterable trait in a particular ethnic group or between ethnic groups such that predicting patient response to a drug is possible, but not necessarily at the present time. Secondly, it could be a characteristic that can be altered reversibly or irreversibly by physiological or pathological factors, often age related, which might include the chronic administration of drugs. Thirdly, it is significantly affected by a wide variety of so-called environmental factors such as diet, but many of the reported differences might be a function of the method of acquisition of the clinical data and their reporting, rather than actual real differences in pathophysiology or biochemistry.

Pharmacokinetic variation

Many of the reported pharmacokinetic variations that might be attributed to ethnic-factors could actually be due to a rather simple overview of the pharmacokinetic indices that we use for comparative purposes and these indices, as discussed by Professor Naito, fail to take into account adequately the physiological factors which might lead to different interpretation, such as weight, body surface area, clearance and so on. But, even if these differences in pharmacokinetic parameters are still apparent, their clinical relevance in routine clinical practice may not be critical. Dr Balant emphasised that we should be careful not to concentrate on what is scientifically fascinating, but rather on what is relevant to the development of a drug and to the health of a patient. However, it would be equally wrong to assume that these differences are not worthy of very detailed evaluation, particularly during the drug development programme.

Drug development programme

If the development process is overburdened with studies that seek to address potential variability, whether it be sub intra-genetic or between ethnic groups, or studies in a wider variety of patient populations, this could have a very major consequence for development times and expense, which would likely be reflected in increases in the cost and therefore the price of medicines. The cost and the implications of the so-called minority data being borne by those whom may be called the majority, are perhaps worthy of further consideration. It has become necessary in health economic terms to look carefully at the cost of drug development and hence the price of drugs; are we to see that change by our desire at this stage to know more about these ethnic parameters?

During early drug development, the emphasis of studies relating to ethnic or genetic factors is largely based upon dose–concentration effects. However, Dr Balant pointed out the importance to the eventual practice of medicine that the Phase III studies concentrate on dose–response parameters. Is medical practice, particularly in the developed world, changing to give us a much more reasonable approach to titrating the patient need against the drug concentration, or are we going to be realistically faced with *"one three times a day for a fortnight and come back and see me if it doesn't work"*? In terms of variation for whichever cause, are we going to become better at more accurately scientifically handling dose–concentration–response affects?

Medical practice

One of the key points from a number of the papers in Session I, was that many of the factors which are loosely described as ethnic differences and discussed without recourse to data, may be related to the methodology used in clinical research rather than real differences, and perhaps the methodology, in turn, is critically dependent upon medical practice. Variations in medical practice are very evident within Europe where medical traditions differ considerably, but has the advent of Good Clinical Research Practice (GCRP) changed that? What formerly was a problem in carrying out extensive clinical evaluations across different countries in Europe is becoming less of a problem now there is a ready acceptance intellectually as well as practically and compliance with GCRP standards. But, in Japan, as pointed out in the review by Dr Hirokawa and Sir Colin Dollery, medical tradition in clinical research practice differs philosophically and practically quite sizeably from those standards currently used in the USA and in Europe. There is an emphasis on safety, with global responses and utility ratings being used. There are large numbers of centres with few patients (typically four per centre), a multiplicity of endpoints, a concentration on reporting severe adverse events, a tendency to minimise or exclude reporting of minor adverse events, and a reluctance to use placebos. Whereas it might have been apparent at the time that these represented a rather superficial evaluation of clinical activity, some also reflected that perhaps the Japanese approach more properly reflects actual practice. The difficulty we face is that this is changing again as a result of the introduction of the 1992 Japanese guidelines, particularly the size of the trials, the use of single primary endpoints, the limitation, hopefully, of the number of centres with an increase in number of patients per centre (although still very small numbers, 4–8), and the need pharmaco-economically to demonstrate superiority. But even then, the process of change for the 1992 guidelines still requires considerable change in the practice of clinical research in Japan, and we must not assume that because a guideline is there, overnight it will become a pattern of activity. By contrast, Drs Edwards and Henderson pointed out the very different socio-historical traditions of medicine and culture in the United States with high science, aggressive activity, the need for public defence of decisions, a confrontational style of activity, and higher risk elements involved in assessments of causes of treatment. This emphasises the enormous gulf between these countries in terms of eventual harmonisation.

So on one hand there is a changing pattern in Japan and on the other hand an established pattern in America and the unification of GCRP in Europe. Those at the First International Conference on Harmonisation (ICH1) in Brussels felt that perhaps ICH3 was the time all of this could come together, but the papers in Session I suggest that the time lines are going to be a little more prolonged. In fact, what key elements of clinical harmonisation are necessary and what elements could be sacrificed if it really was a question of achieving a better degree of communication and use of data?

Harmonisation of requirements

Whereas harmonisation of requirements is a very desirable goal, and the use of data from one geography in another geography a very efficient means of minimising time to market and cost of development, nevertheless from the industrial point of view it is perhaps equally desirable to conduct studies in different populations, and in many different areas of clinical practice. In practical terms, as pointed out by Dr Patterson, obtaining all the data in one country for use in others is not likely to be feasible for several reasons. Firstly, in doing the clinical work in a broad range of geographies we gain a real understanding of the local practice of medicine in that particular area of specialisation. Secondly, this can enable regulators to begin to learn about the products early in the process. The third reason is the positive involvement of local experts and those who therefore will become opinion leaders. The last is the involvement of local company staff and I believe that if multinational, international organisations communicate their new products to local staff at an early stage, they have a much greater commitment, understanding and ability to maximise time to peak sales.

In my opinion, even though harmonisation is a necessary, desirable goal and universal acceptance of data from a wide range of sources an ideal situation, it does not necessarily mean that we will not be conducting studies in a large number of countries. Dr Patterson described how best practice in so-called "globalisation" can be achieved. He gave an interesting analogy with a production process assembly line "driving" the strategic clinical plan from studies into reports, into data to "customers"; whether they be regulators or whether they be physicians, pharmacists or marketing staff. Such an assembly line has inputs from various parts of organisations and external agencies and is a useful way of looking at the clinical process. To Dr Patterson, global does not mean universal, but means a focus on a few key countries, notably the USA, Japan, Germany, France, Italy, the UK and Canada, although to acquire adequate data in the right time, he extended the list to 16 sovereign countries, which for Zeneca now includes Hungary and Czechoslovakia.

Dr Gennery, on the other hand, reflected perhaps the obverse; i.e. the considerable organisational and economic hurdles a Japanese company faces when it tries to globalise and attempts to determine these ethnic or genetic parameters. A particular problem is their lack of marketing intelligence around the world and therefore the pattern of product development and clinical understanding is not well understood by the parent company. Other problems include: cultural gaps of language and business practice; viewing Europe as a single entity or a collection of individual States; an appreciation of the separation of registration needs from those important pricing and reimbursement needs which at times have to come together in clinical studies; and, lastly the very difficult problem of understanding the investment needs and the cost of doing R&D outside Japan which is on a wholly different level to that within Japan.

Session II

THE RELEVANCE OF ETHNIC FACTORS IN THE CLINICAL EVALUATION OF MEDICINES

12
The acceptability of foreign data in the registration of new medicines – Health Protection Branch viewpoint

KATHERINE VOITH

Summary

1. To be acceptable to the Health Protection Branch (HPB) clinical trials must be conducted in accordance with the highest scientific, medical and ethical standards, by an experienced clinician in a reliable medical institution. In foreign clinical trials, the HPB requires assurance that the diagnostic criteria are similar to those used in Canada, that the drug used as a standard is marketed in Canada, and that the rating scales utilised are valid and reliable in both Caucasian and non-Caucasian patients.

2. Canada is reviewing its policy on the inclusion of women in clinical trials, to encourage their participation at an earlier stage of drug development. Furthermore, the HPB proposes that trials submitted to support the use of drugs in the elderly should include patients with an average age closer to that of the clinical population.

3. The quality of data will have a predominant influence on the acceptability of studies; however, data from pharmacokinetic and dose-ranging studies and pivotal clinical trials in the Canadian and North American target population will remain a requirement.

Introduction

The influence of racial differences on the pharmacokinetics, therapeutic effects and toxicity of drugs is a subject of increasing scientific interest. Canada is committed to international harmonisation and the scientific aspects discussed and regulatory positions put forward in these proceedings will be carefully considered by the Health Protection Branch. The conclusions will influence both the pharmaceutical industry and regulatory authorities in the ways they develop and assess new drugs.

The Health Protection Branch (HPB) is one of the eight branches of Health and Welfare Canada, and the Drugs Directorate one of five directorates within the HPB. There are six bureaux within the Drugs Directorate: Dangerous Drugs, Drug Research, Pharmaceutical Surveillance, Nonprescription Drugs, Human Prescription Drugs, and Biologics, the latter three having regulatory roles regarding new therapeutic agents.

Clinical trials accepted by HPB

Most of the clinical trials submitted in Canadian New Drug Submissions (NDS) are conducted in North America and Europe. There seems to be an increase in the number of multicentre studies conducted both in Canada and the US, which is probably due to similarities in language, medical practice, diet, culture, customs and the drug development process. The majority of data are generated in Caucasian populations. Ethnically diverse data may originate from a foreign country, but we do not see enough foreign data to have an impact on our decisions. Ethnic subpopulations enrolled into clinical trials within North America are too small in number to allow for subset-analysis. Consequently, submissions do not contain meaningful efficacy and/or safety data in various ethnic groups.

Table 12.1 outlines the criteria of an acceptable clinical trial. The study must be conducted according to the highest scientific, medical and ethical standards, by an experienced clinician in a reliable medical institution. It should have a clearly defined objective, diagnosis and inclusion and exclusion criteria. Drugs used as standards and their doses should be appropriate, rating scales should be valid and reliable, efficacy parameters should be defined *a priori*, safety should be ensured and the data should lend themselves to statistical analysis. In a foreign clinical trial we would have to ensure that the diagnostic criteria are similar to those used in

Table 12.1 Acceptability of clinical trials – criteria

- Highest scientific, medical and ethical standards
- Experienced clinician
- Reliable medical institution
- Study
  - Objective
  - Diagnostic criteria
  - Inclusion/exclusion criteria
  - Standards (marketed in Canada)
  - Rating scales (cultural influences)
  - Efficacy parameters: *a priori*
  - Safety
  - Statistics

Canada, that the drug used as standard is marketed in Canada and that rating scales utilised are valid and reliable both in Caucasian and non-Caucasian patients.

Effects of ethnicity

There are some examples where ethnicity clearly plays a role. Two recent publications assessed the effect of ethnicity upon the validity and reliability of rating scales. Rating scales used in the assessment of schizophrenia, namely the Positive and Negative Syndrome Scale (PANSS) and the Scales for Assessment of Positive and Negative Symptoms were developed in the 1980s in the US. The Swedish version of the PANSS (von Knorring and Lindstrom, 1992) is a strict translation of the original scale and its validity and reliability were similar to that obtained with the original English language version. The Chinese version of the positive and negative symptom scales introduced some culturally sensitive changes to make definitions more compatible with Chinese professional usage and more consistent with social conditions. Results from a large multicentre study indicated that meaningful comparisons could be made between the original and the Chinese versions (Phillips *et al.*, 1991). Consequently, rating scales established and validated in Western culture must undergo culturally sensitive revision and rigorous evaluation prior to their use in non-Western culture.

I would like to discuss briefly the impact of race and age on antihypertensive therapy. As shown in Table 12.2, in the United States hypertension is more prevalent and has an earlier onset in

Table 12.2 Prevalance of hypertension in the US population*

| Age group | Per cent | | | |
| (years) | Males | | Females | |
	White	Black	White	Black
35–44	26	44	17	37
65–74	59	67	66	83

* Adapted from Weir (1991).

the black population. The incidence of hypertension also increases with age. The underlying haemodynamic mechanism of hypertension varies among black and white and young and old patients and a low renin activity in black patients is a well-established finding. A recent study, conducted in the US by the Department of Veterans Administration, evaluated the comparative effectiveness of six anti-hypertensive drugs which represented the major classes of these agents (Materson *et al.*, 1993). There were 1292 patients in the study, 48% of them black. The results (Table 12.3) indicated that diltiazem, a calcium channel blocker, was the most effective in both young and elderly blacks, while captopril, an ACE inhibitor, was the least effective. Since plasma renin activity is low in black patients, the low efficacy observed with an ACE inhibitor was not surprising. In contrast, in young white patients, captopril was the most effective, while in older whites atenolol produced the best results; captopril was third. The study suggests that in order to optimise

Table 12.3 Single drug therapy for hypertension in white and black men*

Patients	Most effective	Least effective
Blacks:		
Younger (49 yr)	diltiazem	captopril
Older (66 yr)	diltiazem	captopril
Whites:		
Younger (51 yr)	captopril	hydrochlorothiazide
Older (66 yr)	atenolol	prazosin

N=1292 male veterans, 48% black.
Drugs: diltiazem, hydrochorothiazide, clonidine, prazosin, atenolol, captopril, placebo.
* Adapted from Materson *et al.* (1993).

Table 12.4 Ethnic differences in drug disposition*

• Debrisoquine hydroxylation polymorphism	
Poor metabolisers	5–10% Caucasians 1% Chinese, Japanese, Arabic
• Benzodiazapines	
Higher plasma concentrations Lower clearance	Orientals *vs.* Caucasians
• Amobarbital	
Different primary metabolites	Orientals *vs.* Caucasians
• Codeine	
Decreased glucuronidation	Chinese *vs.* Caucasians

* Adapted from Wood and Zhou (1991).

antihypertensive therapy, treatment should be individualised according to the patient's race and age.

Two recent publications indicate that African blacks show a poor response to ACE inhibitors, while in Japanese subjects satisfactory lowering of blood pressure was achieved (Ajayi, 1991; Takabatake *et al.*, 1991). This indicates that low plasma renin activity in blacks is probably genetic since lifestyle, diet, etc. are vastly different between American and African blacks.

Table 12.4 illustrates some examples where drug metabolism is affected by ethnicity. The incidence of poor metabolisers, due to debrisoquine hydroxylation polymorphism, is higher among Caucasians than among other races. Studies indicate that the plasma concentration of benzodiazepines is higher and clearance lower in Orientals when compared to Caucasians. The primary metabolites of amobarbital are different in Caucasians than in Orientals. Codeine glucuronidation is lower in Chinese subjects than in Caucasians.

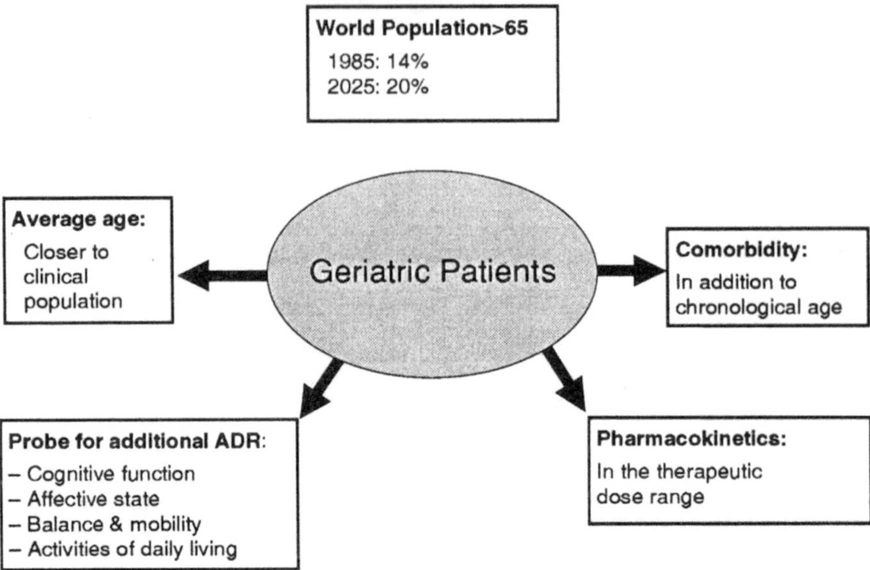

Figure 12.1 Clinical trials to reflect the increasing number of elderly

Females and the elderly in clinical trials

I would like to briefly discuss the position of the Health Protection Branch regarding the participation in clinical trials of two other subpopulations, namely female patients and the elderly. Women, particularly of childbearing potential, are often under represented in clinical trials. For example, more than 95% of the patient population was male in new drug submissions in Canada for potential anti-AIDS drugs. The FDA's recent policy indicates that more women will be included in clinical trials and at an earlier stage of drug development. Canada will most likely adopt a similar policy, since both our in-house experts and clinical investigators support such a policy.

The elderly are the largest consumers of drugs, particularly of those that are indicated for long-term use. The number of elderly is steadily increasing in our societies (Figure 12.1), and in North America, the average nursing home patient is an 86-year-old female. Despite these statistics, the patient population, submitted to support the use of a given drug in the elderly, does not represent the typical elderly patient. We would like to propose that the average age should be closer to that of the clinical population encountered, that comorbidity be considered in addition to chronological age, that

Table 12.5 Conclusions

- Interest in increased foreign content
- Quality of data
- Data required in target populations:
  - Pharmacokinetic studies
  - Dose-ranging studies
  - Pivotal clinical trials
- Future expectations
  - Comparative data from various ethnic groups
  - Discussion of potential differences

cognitive function, affective state, balance and mobility and ability to perform activities of daily living be specifically evaluated in addition to probing adverse drug reactions usually looked at in younger subjects. Pharmacokinetic studies should be carried out in the recommended therapeutic dose range.

Conclusion

In conclusion, the Canadian Health Protection Branch is interested in studies conducted in non-Caucasian populations in order to define inter-ethnic differences and we foresee, that in the future, drug submissions will have increased foreign content (Table 12.5). The quality of data will have a predominant influence on the acceptability of studies. Data in the Canadian and North American target population will remain a requirement. I think of greatest interest will be results that allow meaningful comparisons between different ethnic groups in the effectiveness and safety of new drugs.

I would like to close by quoting from Rutledge (1991) who suggested that industry must face the challenge of acknowledging racial differences in drug response and must enrol and study various racial groups in order to prevent any particular group from becoming a therapeutic orphan.

References

Ajayi AA (1991). Angiotensin converting enzyme inhibitors in cardiovascular and renal disease in Africans: A review. *Afr J Med Sci*, **20**:123–134.

Materson BJ, Rada DJ, Cushman WC *et al*. (1993). Single-drug therapy for hypertension in men. A comparison of six antihypertensive agents with placebo. *N Engl J Med*, **328**:914–921.

Phillips MR, Xiong W, Wang RW *et al.* (1991). Reliability and validity of the Chinese versions of the Scales for Assessment of Positive and Negative symptoms. *Acta Psychiat Scand*, **84**:364–370.

Rutledge DR (1991). Are there beta-adrenergic receptor response differences between racial groups? *DICP*, **25**:824–834.

Takabatake T, Ohta H, Yamamoto Y *et al.* (1991). Effect of atenolol or enalapril on diurnal changes of blood pressure in Japanese mild to moderate hypertensives: A double-blind, randomized, crossover study. *J Hum Hypertens*, **5**:199–204.

von Knorring L and Lindstrom E (1992). The Swedish version of the Positive and Negative Syndrome Scale (PANSS) for schizophrenia. *Acta Psychiat Scand*, **86**:463–468.

Weir MR (1991). Impact of age, race and obesity on hypertensive mechanisms and therapy. *Am J Med*, **90**(Suppl. 5A):3S–14S.

Wood AJJ and Zhou HH (1991). Ethnic differences in drug disposition and responsiveness. *Clin Pharmacokinet*, **20**:350–373.

13
The acceptability of foreign data in the registration of new medicines

Discussants: JENS SCHOU and MARISA PAPALUCA

JENS SCHOU

Danish applications

Being a member of the Licensing Committee, providing recommendations to the Danish National Board of Health, which approves marketing authorisation of new medicines, I would prefer to discuss the topic from a Danish viewpoint.

The Danish Licensing Committee puts special emphasis on controlled clinical trials, and not on open trials, even though large amounts of material from such trials are often presented. The Committee is flexible and liberal in accepting the results of controlled clinical trials from international sources as sufficient evidence, and data from ethnic populations other than Danish are not excluded. However, the Committee prefers studies with patients having been exposed to the drug for which marketing authorisation is being sought under Danish conditions, because of differences in diagnostic and therapeutic traditions for drugs marketed in different areas. Therefore, we prefer data from a controlled clinical study comparing the drug for which marketing authorisation is being sought to a similar medicinal product already marketed in Denmark. We believe this to be the best way to compare a new therapy with a well-known and familiar one. Thus, together with our Scandinavian colleagues, we are different from other members of the European Community.

It is interesting that the authorities in New Zealand do not demand clinical trials on Maori inhabitants, who constitute 30% of the population. Data on a mixed New Zealand population are satisfactory, and it is not required that clinical trials include Maori individuals. They readily extrapolate from the Caucasian and mixed part of the population to the 30% Maoris who, being at a relatively lower social level, possibly represent a major part of the patient population.

Acceptability of non-reactants in the patient population

With regard to the point raised by Dr Voith on the differences in glucuronidation of codeine, I believe that the genetic polymorphism in the demethylation of codeine to morphine is probably more important. In certain populations there are 10% poor metabolisers which do not transform codeine into morphine. When administering codeine, morphine formed by biotransformation is the active drug and codeine should be considered a pro-drug. This means that the poor metabolisers do not receive any effect from codeine. I believe that particularly for very effective and essential drugs, there should be a limit for the acceptability of non-reactants in the population.

Reporting of adverse drug reactions

I am pleased to mention the international activities to obtain standards in the reporting of adverse drug reactions (ADRs). Dr Papaluca and myself have participated in the activities of the CIOMS (Council on International Organizations of Medical Sciences), which has arranged conferences where participants from the industry and regulatory authorities get together in working parties to try to provide recommendations for international use. This activity has already led to two publications, one on the ADR reporting scheme (CIOMS, 1990) and the other on safety updates (CIOMS, 1992). The European Community Pharmacovigilance Working Party is interested in adopting as far as possible the principles given in the CIOMS publications. At present a CIOMS III Working Party is drafting a new publication on the core data sheets, which will be available in 1994. I would like to emphasise the importance of adopting safety evaluation and general ADR reporting problems as a topic for ICH3, as there is an unavoidable link between pre-approval and post-approval experiences when it comes to safety assessment of new medicines.

References

CIOMS (1990). International Reporting of Adverse Drug Reactions. Final Report of CIOMS Working Group. CIOMS, Geneva.

CIOMS (1992). International Reporting of Periodic Drug Safety Update Summaries. Final Report of CIOMS Working Group II. CIOMS, Geneva.

MARISA PAPALUCA

European and Italian viewpoint

In my experience, both in the national evaluation and in the European evaluation of medical dossiers, ethnic differences and the acceptability of data from foreign countries is already a reality in Europe. In the last six months, I reviewed seven clinical dossiers, all of which included information from not only other European countries, but also from the United States and Japan. I am currently following a Multi-State procedure in eight Member States, containing a substantial amount of clinical information derived from Asian populations. When validating this dossier for the European procedure, we tried to take into account previous experiences with the Concertation Procedure. Another example is the registration of a new indication for a known product on the basis of two pivotal studies, one of which was conducted in Japan. Also, one of the dossiers which is now under consideration in Europe, includes the new approach of incorporating a pharmacokinetic (PK) screen analysis in order to improve the interpretation of pharmacokinetic data.

As far as Italy is concerned, we are now reviewing dossiers containing a substantial amount of non-European, non-Caucasian data. In the past we demanded that clinical trials be conducted in Italy before an application, but during the last three or four years the attitude has changed considerably. Taking into account the European regulations, we now have to accept data from clinical trials performed in other Member States, even with comparators which are not on the market in Italy. We do therefore accept data from comparative trials with products which have not been used in Italy.

Application of foreign data

In principle, there is no clinical data which is not reviewed, and there is no useful information which is not utilised independently from its origin. This is true for Italy, and for Europe at least as far as my experience of the last three years is concerned. However, the weight attached to the information received from third parties depends very much on the application. It is much easier for us to interpret studies carried out in the USA because there is a longer experience and many standards have been homogenised. On the other hand, we have received in recent years, substantial numbers of patients from Japan. For example, in a dossier I reviewed recently 2300 patients were exposed in Japan, and in our opinion very important information can be derived from these patients because human beings are the same everywhere in the world. When we receive data which are not, as we would normally define them, really pivotal, we use it as supporting data. This does not mean the importance is diminished because, for example, there is now a tendency for many companies to reduce the size of double blind randomised trials and the time of follow up in order to reduce costs. Therefore, if 2000 patients are exposed, safety data from an additional 2000 patients is quite important to have. It is not just supportive in the generic sense, but may demonstrate that even in groups completely different from our own, there is a good tolerability and a declared efficacy of the product. So I think we are in this sense already anticipating the future.

Problems in reviewing foreign data

The problem that reviewers have, particularly in reviewing the safety data from large numbers of patients studied in Japan, for example, relates to the fact that in certain cases we are not sure that the side-effects refer to a patient that was properly enrolled. I believe that in order to speed up and to ameliorate the acceptability of foreign data, particularly data from the Asian area and Japan, it is very important for the companies to begin to address these problems, rather than simply waiting for the harmonisation of the rules. It is desirable to have, for example, the Japanese data presented according to the Japanese way. In my experience each company tends to present data from other areas in the same format as they present data from the US or other countries in Europe. Transferring Japanese experiences to European or American models makes it difficult to understand what is behind the data and to extrapolate the results. As we know, there are differences in the diagnostic criteria, in study design and so on, and when the data are presented in a classical way, we are not confident and we have to go back to the single patient data, which wastes time in the review procedure.

What Professor Schou said is correct. Usually, in Europe, we believe that it is desirable to include classical double blind controlled studies in a dossier, even for populations which are outside Europe or the USA. But I know that sometimes in Japan it is not possible to carry out this kind of study, and I think that the best way is to present the data as they are and not to try to convert them and give explanations. Certain pieces of information are missing in dossiers when data from abroad is reported. For example, for an antitubercular drug which I reviewed, for which substantial data came from Asia, there was no information about aspects which could cause large differences, such as the lifestyle of the patients, if they were rural, living in big cities, the kind of education. We have been speaking about ethnicity, about genotyping patients and so on, but I think that particularly for the so-called efficacy studies it is important to have details on how those people are living. If we do not have this information we cannot evaluate the data properly.

If we want to resolve the problem of racial differences, we have to try to understand what is happening in general terms, as we are doing in this seminar and in the ICH process, but also in particular when we receive the actual data, to see what the problems are and to try to resolve them case by case in parallel with the general discussions.

14
Ethnic effects on pharmacokinetic parameters

CHIKAYUKI NAITO

Summary

1. So-called ethnic differences in the efficacy and safety of drugs have been a major hindrance for the mutual acceptance of foreign clinical data. The Japanese Ministry of Health and Welfare therefore analysed pharmacokinetic parameters for the same medicines approved in different countries, in order to assess genetic influences on drug metabolism.

2. The results obtained from comparing mean values for different populations suggest that so-called ethnic differences might be influenced by environmental rather than genetic factors. However, examination of mean data may be inappropriate to elucidate ethnic profiles of drug metabolism, and individual pharmacokinetic data have also been assessed.

3. Although the data are limited at present, the inter-ethnic differences do not seem to be larger than the intra-ethnic variations. These results suggest that foreign pharmacokinetic data from Phase I studies, if performed properly, could be utilised mutually irrespective of the differences in race.

Introduction

So-called ethnic differences in the efficacy and safety of drugs have been a major hindrance for the mutual acceptance of foreign clinical data.

Table 14.1 Differences in approved dosage of deliberately selected drugs used in Japan, USA and EC

	Daily dose		
Drugs	*Japan*	*USA*	*EC*
Antihypertensives:			
Captopril	37.5–75 mg	50–150 mg	12.5–150 mg
Celiprolol HCl	100–200 mg	—	200–400 mg
Cilazapril	0.5–2 mg	2.5–5 mg	2.5–5 mg
Doxazosin mesylate	1–4 mg	1–10 mg	1–16 mg
Enalapril maleate	5–10 mg	10–40 mg	10–40 mg
Metoprolol tartrate	60–120 mg	100–450 mg	50–400 mg
Terazosin HCl	1–4 mg	1–5 mg	2–10 mg
Anti-arrhythmics:			
Flecainide acetate	100–200 mg	300–400 mg	100–400 mg
Mexiletine HCl	300–450 mg	600–900 mg	600–800 mg
Propafenone HCl	450 mg	150–450 mg	450–900 mg
Antibiotics:			
Clarithromycin	400 mg	375 mg	500–1000 mg
Imipenem cilastatine	0.5–1 g	1–4 g	1–4 g
Antibacterials:			
Ciprofloxacin HCl	200–600 mg	500–1000 mg	—
Enoxacin	200–600 mg	400–800 mg	400–800 mg
Ofloxacin	300–600 mg	400–800 mg	200–800 mg
Antiviral:			
Acyclovir	1000 mg	600–1200 mg	4000 mg
Antihistamines:			
Terfenadine	60 mg	60–120 mg	120 mg
Psychotropics:			
Lormetazepam	1–2 mg	—	0.5–1.5 mg
Triazolam	0.25 mg	0.25–0.5 mg	—
Anti-inflammatory:			
Nabumetone	800 mg	1500–2000 mg	1000 mg
Tenoxicam	10–20 mg	20–40 mg	20 mg

There are differences between Japan and the West in the approved daily dosages of many drugs (Table 14.1); however such differences can also be found between the USA and the EC. Further comparisons of both the maximum and minimum approved doses (plotted as a ratio, dose in Japan/foreign dose) for drugs belonging to five therapeutic classes (non-steroidal anti-inflammatory/analgesics, antipsychotics, cardiovascular, gastrointestinal and antibiotics) that have been developed in countries other than Japan, and have also been approved in Japan, have been carried out. These show that there are no apparent differences in the doses approved in Japan and in foreign countries, judged by the average ratio for each therapeutic class for both maximum and minimum approved doses (Figure 14.1). However, closer evaluation of the data shows that for the non-steroidal anti-inflammatory/analgesics and antibiotics the approved doses in Japan tend to be lower than in other countries for both the minimum and maximum approved dose, while for cardiovascular drugs the Japanese dose in the maximum range seems to be lower than in other countries. These differences

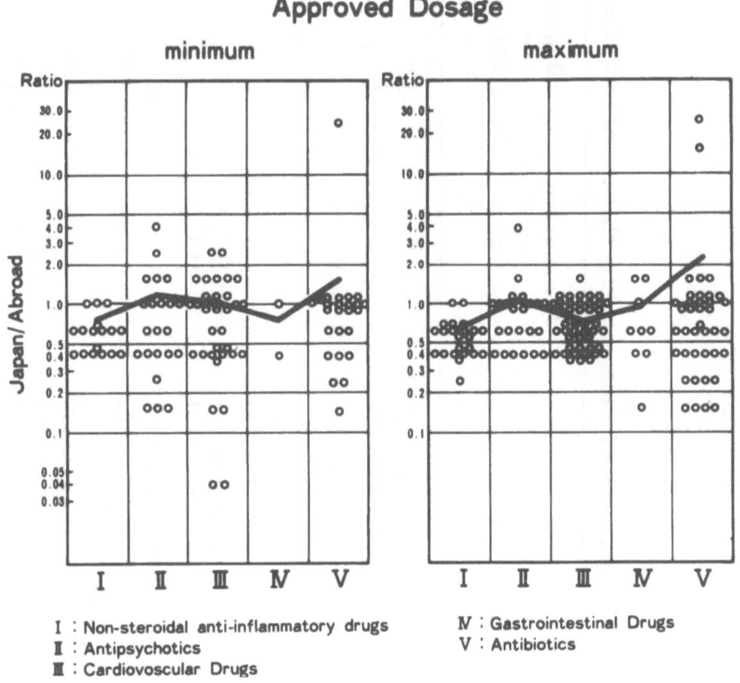

Figure 14.1 Ratio of approved dosage in Japan and other countries (By courtesy of Dr Shimizu). Reproduced from Naito (1992) with permission.

Table 14.2 Comparison of pharmacokinetic parameters of approved antibiotics among different countries

Name of drugs		Pharmacokinetics in healthy volunteers (single-dose study)					
		Dose	C_{max} (µg)	T_{max} (min)	$T^{1/2}$ (h)	*AUC* (µg.hr/ml)	*Urinary excretion* (%)
CZX	Japanese	0.5 g im (*n*=6)	18.66	45.6	1.39	56.17	Ca. 90 (0–24 hr)
	USA	0.5 g im (*n*=8)	13.7	54	1.42	55.3	Ca. 80 (0–8 hr)
COZM	Japanese	0.5 g iv (*n*=4)	100.9		2.32	173	78.61±13.65
	USA	0.5 g iv (*n*=6)	133±9		2.4±0.5	251±51	94±10
	Japanese	1.0 g iv (*n*=4)	168.9		2.63	338	90.85±2.98
	USA	1.0 g iv (*n*=12)	215±35		2.5±0.3	426±65	80±8
	Japanese	2.0 g iv (*n*=4)	424.0		2.32	779	83.19±6.99
	USA	2.0 g iv (*n*=12)	394±49		2.5±0.3	790±142	79±7
SCE	Japanese	1.0 g iv (*n*=3)		(hr)	1.56±0.16	161±33	86.3
	German	1.0 g iv (*n*=12)	97.3±25.6	0.08±0.00	1.71±0.19	124±20.3	84.5
	Japanese	2.0 g iv (*n*=3)			1.83±0.14	309±24	92.9
	German	2.0 g iv (*n*=12)	167±51.9	0.15±0.09	2.05±0.27	295±52.0	80.5
	Japanese	0.5 g im (*n*=3)	14.0±0.7		3.10±0.63	85.8±7.7	83.7
	German	0.5 g im (*n*=12)	16.5±5.58	1.08±1.01	2.36±0.5	62.3±7.7	64.9

CEF	Japanese	250 mg im (*n*=14)	9.4±0.7	42.9±3.1	27 (min)	8.9	71.7±3.6	
	UK	250 mg im (*n*=4)	5.2~8.6	30~75			74	
	Japanese	500 mg im (*n*=14)	15.3±1.2	54.6±5.6	31	18.7	74.2±2.0	
	UK	500 mg im (*n*=2)	8.0~10	30~75			69	
	UK	500 mg im (*n*=10)	11.51	30~90	40		72	
ROXI	Japanese	150 mg im (*n*=12)	4.4±2.08	1.4±1.39	6.99±3.15	49.5±20.47 (0–24 hr)	6.76±12.89	
	USA	150 mg im (*n*=20)	6.78±1.16	1.91±1.16	8.38±4.17	70.82±20.01 (0–48 hr)	11.5±4.2	
	Japanese	300 mg im (*n*=12)	7.4±2.42	2.5±2.08	7.90±2.70	97.6±38.45 (0–24 hr)	7.88±12.68	
	USA	300 mg im (*n*=20)	9.11±1.67	1.90±1.30	10.46±5.17	113.55±23.82 (0–48 hr)	10.4±3.3	
ROX	Japanese	0.5 g iv (*n*=4)			6.01	683.5	49.0±12	(0–48 hr)
	USA	0.5 g iv (*n*=12)			6.30	551±91	41±8	(0–48 hr)
	Swiss	0.5 g iv (*n*=6)			7.7±1.2	846±179	64.3±7.3	(0–48 hr)
	Japanese	1.0 g iv (*n*=5)			6.56	1164.9	50.4±2.9	(0–48 hr)
	USA	1.0 g iv (*n*=12)			6.13	1006±118	39±5	(0–48 hr)
CLIN	Japanese	300 mg im (*n*=6)	3.1	1.0	2.7		19.1	(0–6 hr)
	USA	300 mg im (*n*=8)	5.61			36.63		
	Japanese	600 mg im (*n*=6)	4.8	1.0	3.5		11.8	(0–6 hr)
	USA	600 mg im (*n*=6)	5.28			38.1		

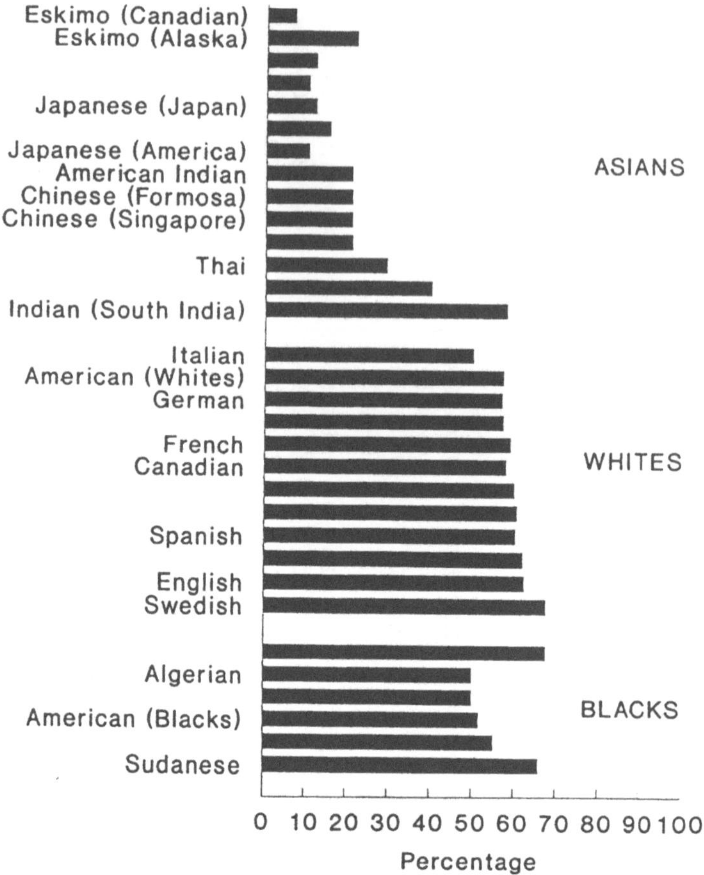

Figure 14.2 Distribution of slow acetylators of isoniazid in different populations (By courtesy of Dr Sunahara).(Reproduced from Naito (1992) with permission)

may be derived from a sort of ethnic difference, which includes both genetic and environmental factors.

The metabolism of isoniazid, which is used in the treatment of tuberculosis, is greatly influenced by genetic factors. Following ingestion, isoniazid is subjected to acetylation and is excreted in the urine. Its metabolic rate varies widely from individual to individual and there are roughly two populations, rapid acetylators and slow acetylators. The distribution of rapid and slow acetylators is notably different from nation to nation (Figure 14.2). For example, about 60% of all Caucasians are slow acetylators while only about 10% of all Japanese are slow acetylators. Apart from the classical example of isoniazid, many genetic variants have recently been discovered in relation to drug metabolism, and their clinical significance clarified. However, in order to remove a hindrance to harmonisation arising from genetic factors, it is important to know the degree of the differences between the inter- and intra-ethnic variations, and the proportion of poor and extensive metabolisers in a given race.

Ministry of Health and Welfare study

In order to acquire basic information concerning genetic influences on drug metabolism the Japanese Ministry of Health and Welfare analysed pharmacokinetic parameters for the same medicines approved in different countries. These were obtained from single-dose studies in healthy volunteers and include C_{max}, T_{max}, $T_{1/2}$ AUC and urinary excretion data. All data were expressed as the mean $\pm$ standard deviation (SD) or standard error (SE) for this analysis.

No significant differences were found in pharmacokinetic parameters between Japanese and Caucasians for a cohort of antibiotics (Table 14.2) or antihypertensives (Table 14.3) studied. However, large differences in the approved dosage and the occurrence of adverse events existed for the antihypertensives between Japanese and Caucasians (Table 14.3). These results suggest that so-called ethnic differences might be influenced by environmental rather than genetic factors.

It has been well established that the metabolism of many drugs is catalysed by specific cytochrome P450 enzymes, the activity of which is under genetic rather than environmental control. Therefore, an examination of the pharmacokinetics of drugs whose metabolism is extensively related to that of debrisoquine/sparteine and of mephenytoin was undertaken. UL-O1, an antiulcerant, the metabolism of which is known to be related to the metabolism of mephenytoin gives quite different mean values for AUC and C_{max} between Japanese and Swedish healthy volunteers (Table 14.4). Moreover, the standard deviations of these values were large, suggesting a wide distribution of individual values or the existence of some outliers.

Some differences in pharmacokinetic parameters between Japanese and American healthy volunteers and a skewed distribution of individual values or the existence of some outliers were also seen with ART-FL, an anti-arrythmic drug, of debrisoquine/ sparteine type metabolism (Table 14.5). However, it is realised that the examination of data expressed in terms of mean $\pm$ SD or SE might be inappropriate to elucidate actual ethnic profiles of drug metabo-

Table 14.3 Comparison of pharmacokinetic parameters of approved antihypertensives among different countries

Name of drugs		Pharmacokinetics in healthy volunteer (single-dose study)					Clinical study		
		Dose	C_{max}	T_{max}	$T^{1/2}$	AUC		Dose	ADR
Aten.	JPN	50 mg (n=10)	0.166±0.0126	3	(10.4±2.38)	—	JPN	50 mg*	17.3%
	UK	(200 mg (n=5))	(1.10±0.782)	3	(6.36±0.55)		UK	50~200	—
	USA	50 mg (n=12)	0.282±0.088	3.3±1.3	7.4±0.84	2.65±0.594			
Carvi.	JPN	20 mg (n=5)	53.1	0.9	8.3	233			
	DEU	25 mg (n=19)	55	0.93	6.0	234			
Pind.	JPN	20 mg	50±14.14	2	5.4±0.56	567±172.5			
	SW	20 mg	48.8±16.2	1	8.4±2.0	—			
Bena	JPN	10 mg (n=5)	195.3	0.4	0.5	173.4	JPN	5~20	14.2
	USA	10 mg (n=60)	132.7±48.0	0.5(median)	0.6±0.2	132.7±46.3	SW	20~40	20
Enal	JPN	10 mg (n=6)	103.2	1.7	8.4	663.5	JPN	2.5~10	8.7
	USA	10 mg (n=6)	90.4	1.6	—	682	UK	5~20	28.6
Tera	JPN	1 mg (n=6)	40.4±9.8	1.0	18.70±10.60	580.3±106.1	JPN	0.5~4	13.3
	USA	1 mg (n=18)	19.6	1.0	12.0		USA	1~20	20.1
Doxa	JPN	2 mg (n=6)	18.8±2.0	1.74±2.0	10.14±3.32	233.3±32.5	JPN	0.5~4	15.1
	USA	1 mg (n=24)	(10.1±3.0)	(2.2±1.0)	(11.0±3.0)		USA	1~16	23.4
	UK	2 mg (n=18)	12.9±4.1	2.3±1.0	—	113.1±45.2	USA		48.3
Cila	JPN	5 mg (n=6)	104.1±25.71	2.0±0.55	1.7±0.27	0.345±0.080	JPN	2.5~10	16.9
	UK	5 mg (n=6)	74±29	—	1.6±0.5	0.28±0.02	UK	25~50	15.5

* Open study

Table 14.4 Comparison of pharmacokinetic parameters of an antiulcerant (UL-O1) among different countries (subject: healthy volunteer; route: oral, single admin.; mean±SD)

Country	Dose	N	AUC (ng.h/ml)	C_{max} (ng/ml)	T_{max} (h)	$T\frac{1}{2}$ (h)	Remark
Japan	20 mg	6	1413±1693	517.6±564.8	1.8±1.6	2.2	Mephenytoin type
Sweden	20 mg	12	533.4±915.3	220.3±175.2	1.8±0.7	?	Mephenytoin type

Table 14.5 Comparison of pharmacokinetic parameters of an anti-arrhythmic (ART-F1) among different countries (subject: healthy volunteer; route: oral, single admin.; range (mean))

Country	Dose	N	V_d (l/kg)	$T\frac{1}{2}$ (h)	CLR (ml/min/kg)	Ae (%)*	Remark
Japan	25–250 mg	12	5.5–15.3(8.7)	6.0–14.0(11.0)	5.7–18.5(9.5)	16.2–51.2(33.5)	Debrisoquine type
USA	60–240 mg	16		6.9–22.0(14.2)	4.1–13.7(7.9)	9.9–44.0(24.4)	Debrisoquine type

*Ae: Amount of drug excreted in the urine

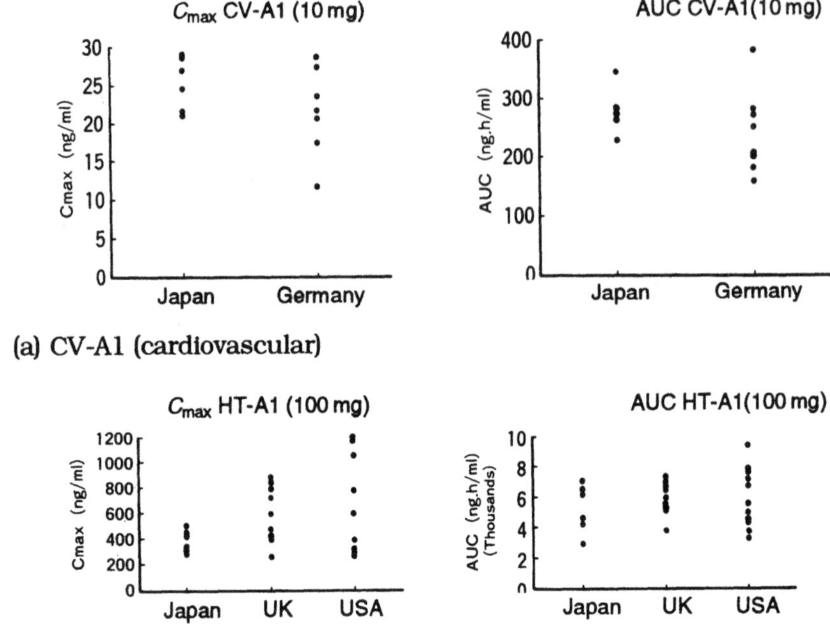

(a) CV-A1 (cardiovascular)

(b) HT-A1 (antihypertensive)*

Figure 14.3 Distribution of C_{max} and AUC in individual subjects.
* Japan & UK: tablets; USA: solution

lism and the analyses of individual pharmacokinetic data of medicines might produce much more reliable and useful information.

Individual pharmacokinetic parameters

A retrospective survey was performed in which individual pharmacokinetic data were collected for certain drugs which were approved or under development between 1985 and the present (1993) in the three geographical regions, USA, Japan and Europe. The AUC, C_{max}, T_{max}, $T_{1/2}$ and urinary excretion data from a single-dose administration, and on day one and the day steady state was achieved in the repeated-dose administration, were examined. Data was collected on about 80 medicines directly from pharmaceutical companies. However, comparison of all parameters on every drug could not be made because several parameters were missing and the administered doses in many cases differed among countries.

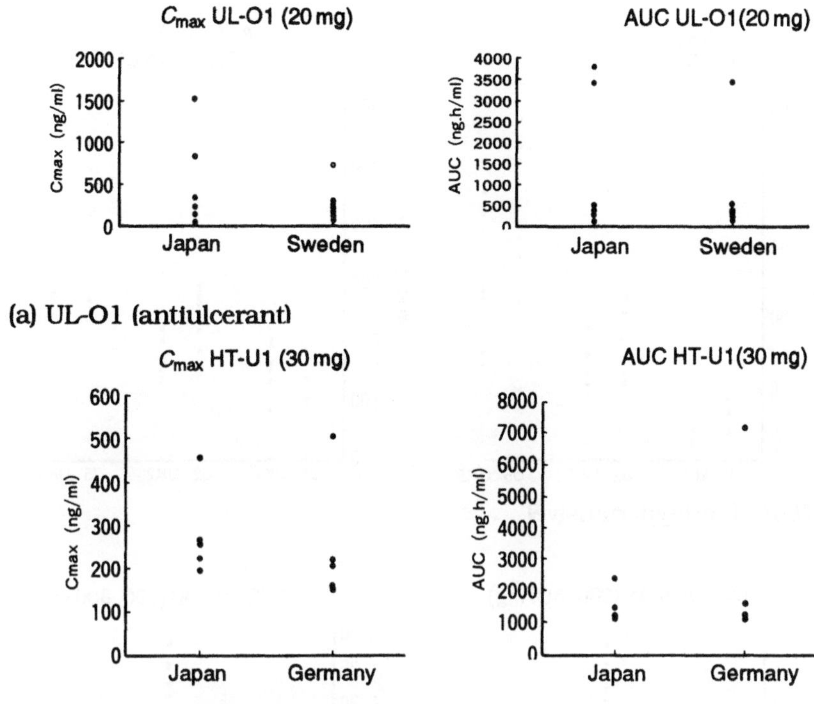

Figure 14.4 Distribution of C_{max} and AUC in individual subjects

Single-dose administration

The values of AUC and C_{max} from the available data for each country were plotted since these parameters are the most relevant to the effect of the medicine. Even when individual values are plotted in most of the medicines examined no significant differences in AUC and C_{max} between Japanese and Caucasians were found as demonstrated by the examples shown in Figure 14.3.

In the case of UL-O1, an antiulcerant which undergoes mephenytoin type metabolism and gives a large standard deviation of the mean values for kinetic parameters in healthy volunteers (Table 14.4), when C_{max} and AUC were plotted as individual points, two outliers were found in Japanese and one in Swedish volunteers (Figure 14.4). This figure also shows that extraordinarily high values of AUC and C_{max} were observed in one or two subjects when individual data were plotted for Japanese and German subjects for

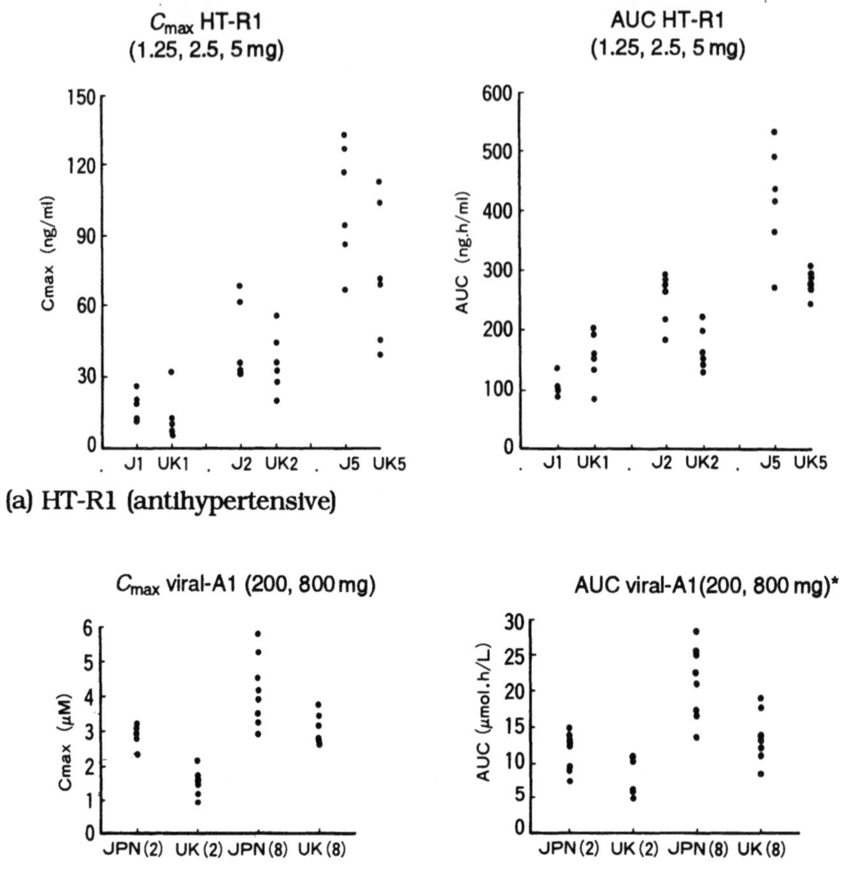

Figure 14.5 Distribution of C_{max} and AUC in individual subjects (Key: J1 = Japan 1.25 mg, UK5 = UK 5 mg; JPN (2) = Japan 200 mg etc.)
*Japan: 0–24 hours, UK: 0–12 hours

an antihypertensive (HT-U1). These results suggest the occurrence of pharmacogenetic defects of P450 enzymes in some individuals.

In the cases of HT-R1, an antihypertensive, and Viral-A1, an antiviral (Figure 14.5), although no outliers are seen, the mean C_{max} and AUC at the higher doses seems greater in Japanese subjects than in British subjects. However, if the AUC and C_{max} values are adjusted by body weight this difference between Japanese and Western subjects may disappear as demonstrated by the distribution of AUC and C_{max} (Figure 14.6) for another antihypertensive (HT-C1).

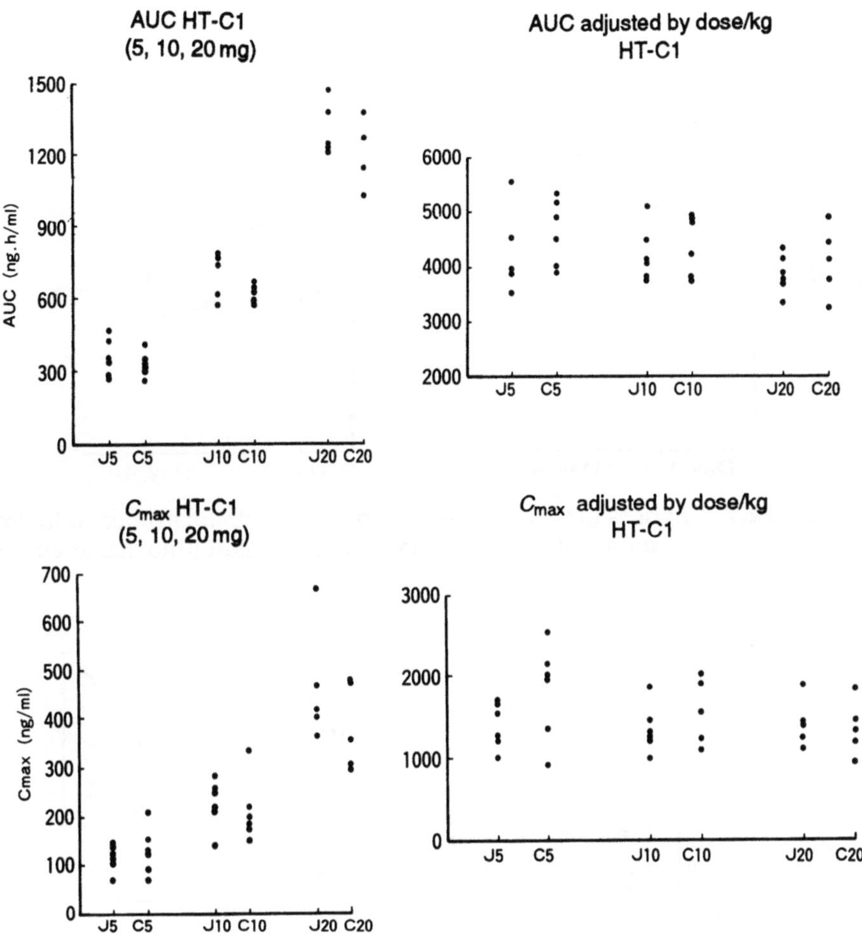

Figure 14.6 Distribution of C_{max} and AUC for HT-C1 (antihypertensive) in individual subjects. (Key: J5 = Japanese 5 mg, C5 = Caucasian 5 mg etc.)

Repeat-dose administration

When this retrospective analysis was initiated it was expected that pharmacokinetic parameters might be similar when steady state was achieved in the repeat-dose administration of a compound as compared to pharmacokinetic parameters from single-dose administration. Contrary to this expectation, the C_{max} increased but the AUC was almost constant after repeated administration for some antibiotics in American subjects (Figure 14.7), whilst in the case of other antibiotics the C_{max} was almost constant but the AUC increased after repeated administration of the compounds (Figure 14.8). For a further cohort of antibiotics, C_{max} tended to increase

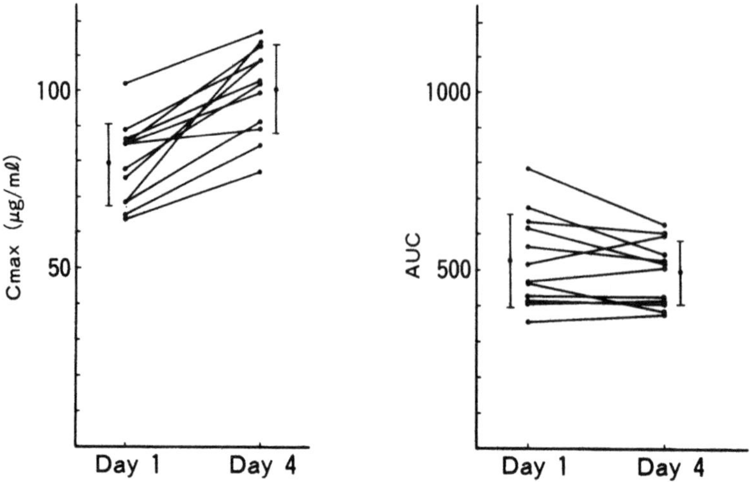

Figure 14.7 Changes in C_{max} and AUC by repeated administration (infusion for 30 min, twice a day) of some antibiotics in American (Caucasian except one Black) volunteers

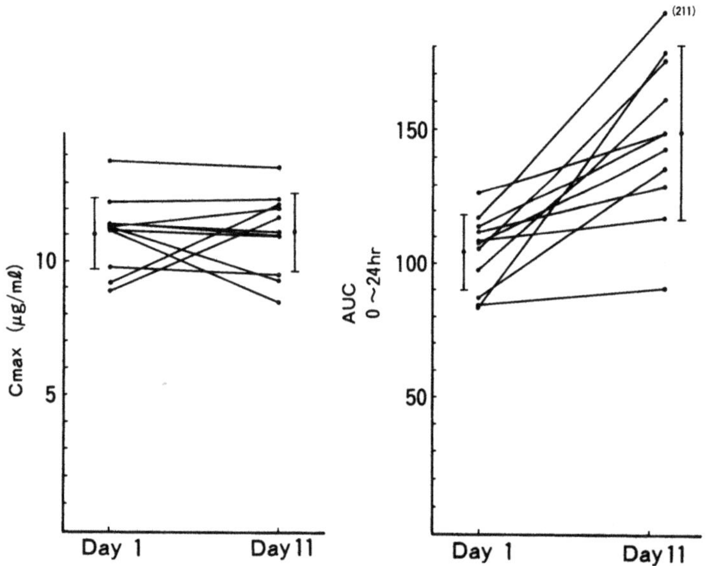

Figure 14.8 Changes in C_{max} and AUC by repeated administration (oral, 300 mg q.d.) of some antibiotics in Caucasian volunteers

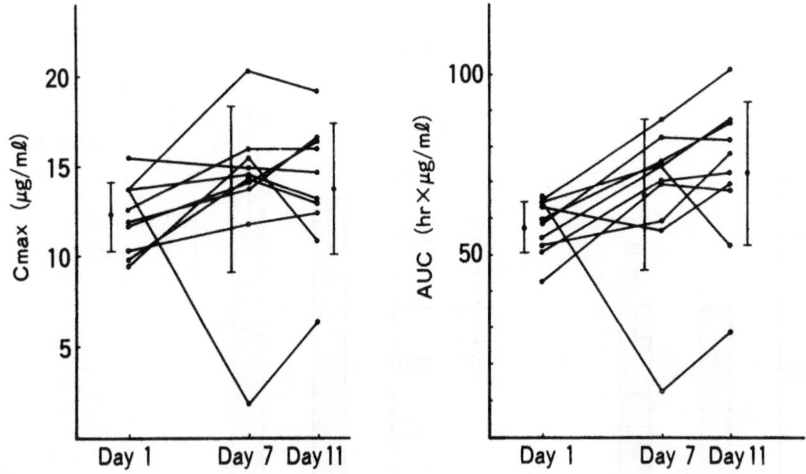

Figure 14.9 Changes in C_{max} and AUC by repeated administration (oral, 300 mg b.i.d.) of some antibiotics in Caucasian volunteers

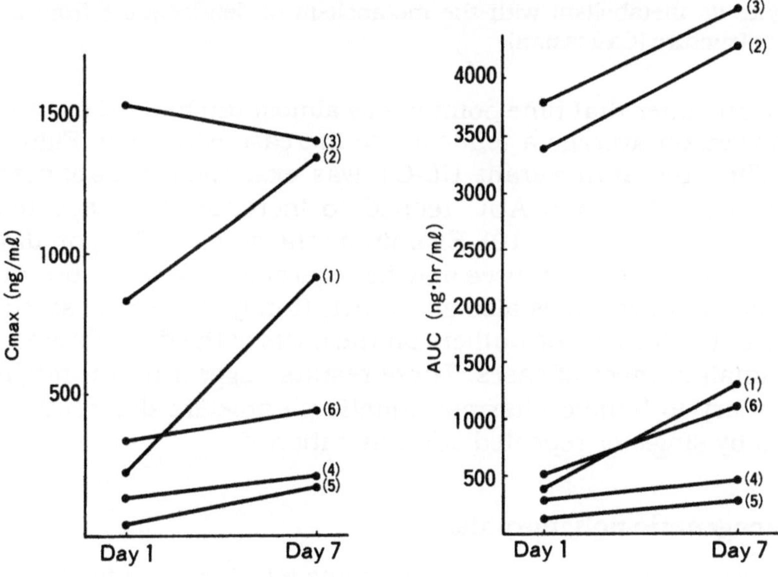

Figure 14.10 Changes in C_{max} and AUC by repeated administration of UL-O1 (antiulcerant) in Japanese volunteers

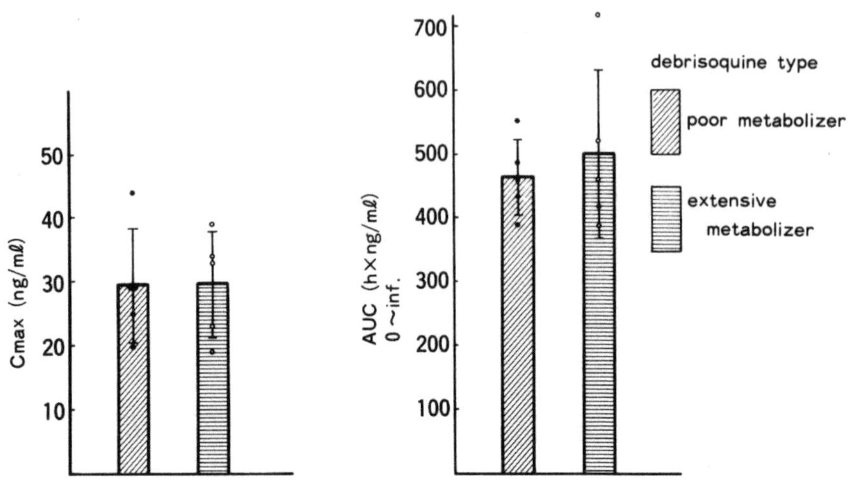

Figure 14.11 C_{max} and AUC of some β-blocker which was suspected to cosegregate its metabolism with the metabolism of debrisoquine from its chemical structure (Caucasian)

on day 7 and after that time point it was almost unchanged but the AUC showed on average a tendency to increase with time (Figure 14.9). When the antiulcerant UL-O1 was examined in Japanese subjects both C_{max} and AUC tended to increase after repeated administration (Figure 14.10). Examining the data for C_{max} on day 1, case numbers two and three may be regarded as outliers, but on day 7 case number one is also an outlier. It may, therefore, sometimes be difficult to define outliers on the basis of the data obtained from a small number of cases. These results suggest that it might be necessary to handle pharmacokinetic parameters differently if obtained by single or repeated administration.

Pharmacogenetic polymorphism

It is well known that a specific cytochrome P450 enzyme is able to oxidise drugs that are not closely related structurally to the prototype substance. This being the case, it is not possible to decide whether or not the metabolism of a given drug is influenced by pharmacogenetic polymorphism by only the likeness of chemical structure. This is demonstrated by a β-blocker which, in spite of a similar chemical structure to other β-blockers with metabolism intimately related to the metabolism of debrisoquine/sparteine, showed no difference in the values of both C_{max} and AUC between poor metabolisers and extensive metabolisers of debrisoquine/ sparteine (Figure 14.11). Furthermore, Wood and Zhou (1991) have reported that the metabolism of propranolol was significantly more extensive in Chinese than in Caucasians but the dynamic response was found to be higher in Chinese subjects than in Caucasians. This report suggests that the pharmacodynamic response cannot always be deduced from pharmacokinetic parameters.

Conclusion

In general, daily dosages of medicines seem to be lower in Japanese than in Caucasians, but judging from the values of AUC and C_{max} for most of the medicines examined, on average, there is no evidence that Japanese subjects can only metabolise drugs more slowly than Caucasians. Although the data are still limited at present, the inter-ethnic differences do not seem to be larger than the intra-ethnic variations. These results suggest that foreign pharmacokinetic data from Phase I studies, if performed properly, could be utilised mutually, irrespective of the differences in race.

Acknowledgement

The author gratefully acknowledges the support of Professor H. Yasuhara and Dr E. Uchida for calculation and analysis of the collected data. The author also expresses his hearty thanks to industries that willingly provided their precious data.

References

Naito C (1992). Some problems relating to dose response trials. In: D'Arcy PF and Harron DWG (eds) *Proceedings of The First International Conference on Harmonisation, Brussels 1991*. The Queen's University of Belfast, pp. 495–511

Wood, AJJ and Zhou, HH (1991). Ethnic differences in drug disposition and responsiveness. *Clin Pharmacokinet*, **20(5)**:350–373

15

A comparison of the clinical evaluation of medicines in Japanese and Caucasian populations

ETIENNE LABBE

Summary

1. In order to compare inter- and intra-ethnic variability in drug response, in Japanese and Caucasian subjects, the clinical data for five drugs has been reviewed, focusing on the pharmacokinetic parameters. These drugs represent different pharmacological/therapeutic classes.

2. No pharmacogenetically linked differences between Caucasian and Japanese subjects were found. With regard to pharmacokinetic parameters, for all five drugs the intra-ethnic variability was higher than the inter-ethnic variability.

3. Differences in methodology and the number of subjects studied might contribute to the apparent variations in pharmacokinetic parameters. In order to draw firm conclusions regarding inter-ethnic differences in drug response it will therefore be necessary to harmonise the principles and technical aspects of drug development methodology.

Ethnic differences in the field of drug evaluation obviously involve many factors linked to the intrinsic characteristics of the individuals – mainly genetic factors – and to extrinsic parameters which could be qualified as cultural and environmental. These include climatic conditions, nutritional behaviour, medical culture, and many othrs. In order to determine whether or not there is an "ethnic effect" on drug response, one approach is to compare the inter-ethnic to the intra-ethnic variability of the drug response.

We conducted a retrospective review of clinical data concerning drugs developed in Western countries and in Japan, focusing on the pharmacokinetic parameters (mainly C_{max} and AUC) which allow the comparison of absorption and drug availability as a function of time in both populations. Five drugs were found to be eligible for such a comparison; three others could not be taken into account since they were developed before 1984–85 and individual data or other important information were not always available. However, statistical analysis could not be performed for these five drugs, since the necessary conditions for test application were not fulfilled.

H_1 receptor antagonist

The first example is taken from the pharmacokinetic data concerning a non-sedative H_1 receptor antagonist under development in Europe and Japan. Six studies were performed in Europe with 18–24 subjects per trial and five studies in Japan with six subjects per trial. The same daily dose was administered in each study. Considering C_{max}, the range of individual data varies by about 30% in both regions but the means are exactly the same. With regard to T_{max} and half-life, the values are around 15% higher in Japanese, but the sampling times were slightly different. As for AUC, the general mean is 12.5% higher in the Japanese which might be related to the body weight difference (63 kg for the Japanese, 72 kg for the Europeans), but the range of individual data is similar. In a specific European study in 24 subjects, the coefficient of variation for AUC and C_{max} were found to be 5.7% and 10.4%, respectively, for intra-subject and 21.7% and 14.4%, respectively, for inter-subect variability.

The pharmacodynamic data under the same test conditions show optimal and similar results in both populations for the same dose given once daily. Safety should be further studied but preliminary results show no particular difference. It can be concluded for this drug that intra-ethnic variability of the pharmacokinetic data is higher than the inter-ethnic variability and that there is no difference in drug response between Caucasian and Japanese.

Antiepileptic agent

For another compound, an antiepileptic drug acting on the $GABA_A$ macromolecular complex, human pharmacokinetic studies were conducted in Europe, Japan and the US; unfortunately only part of the US data were available. This compound is rapidly absorbed and metabolised, yielding an acid which is an active metabolite. Both parent drug and metabolite were studied with regard to the kinetic profile. For the same dose, T_{max}, C_{max} and the elimination half-life are compatible in the three areas, even though the $T_{1/2}$ shows a lower value for the parent drug in the US. However, the US data were judged to be consistent with the European results. $AUC_{0-\infty}$

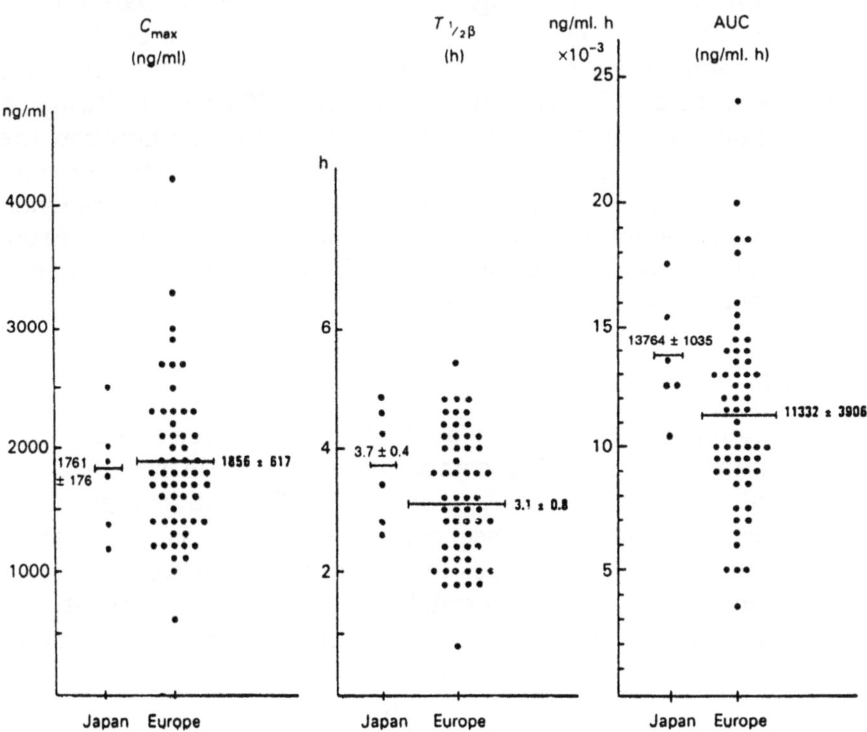

Figure 15.1 Antiepileptic agent. Individual variation of C_{max}, $T_{1/2\beta}$ and AUC values after the administration of 600 mg *per os* to 58 European and six Japanese healthy volunteers

Table 15.1 Hypnotic: Pharmacokinetic data after the administration of 10 mg in three single-dose studies (SD, mean values ± SEM and ranges)

	C_{max}	T_{max}	$T_{1/2\beta}$	$AUC_{0-\infty}$	U recovery 0–24
Europe (n=20)	(130) 139±53 55–222	(1.3) 1.0±0.8 0.3–3.0	(2.4) 1.5±0.6 0.7–3.6	(498) 362±225 82.0–834	0.10
USA (n=30)	100±7.5 39–194	1.36±0.2 0.5–4.0	2.29±0.16 0.83–4.72	427.9±48 88–1035	
Japan (n=6) (s.d.)	119.5±72.9 60.3–261.3	0.8±0.3 0.5–1.0	2.3±1.48 1.11–5.21	491±474 132–1417	0.14

*Numbers in parentheses show values issued from a mathematical model.

mean value is around 20% higher in the Japanese compared to the European data. It is difficult to say if this difference is clinically relevant or not, and it might be related to the body weight difference which is around 20% lower in the Japanese (61 versus 72 kg). A more significant question, however, is the difference between the number of subjects studied as it is inaccurate to compare the data of 58 European subjects to those of six Japanese volunteers when attempting to evaluate inter-subject variability (Figure 15.1). From these available data, no obvious inter-ethnic difference can be seen between Japanese and Caucasian.

Hypnotic

A third example is an hypnotic developed in the three regions. One main characteristic of this compound is the wide range of the individual data concerning C_{max} and AUC. This rather high intra-ethnic variability has been observed in the three areas, contrasting with the narrow range of doses for an optimal response: 5–10 mg. In an attempt to explain the variability of plasmatic concentrations, an identification of the P_{450} isoenzymes involved in the drug metabolism was performed. The results show that several forms are responsible for the hepatic catabolism but no one exclusively, thus a polymorphism of the metabolism can be excluded.

The ranges of C_{max} and AUC values for different studies have been plotted, showing comparable means and maximum/minimum values in the three regions (Table 15.1). Once again, for one dose,

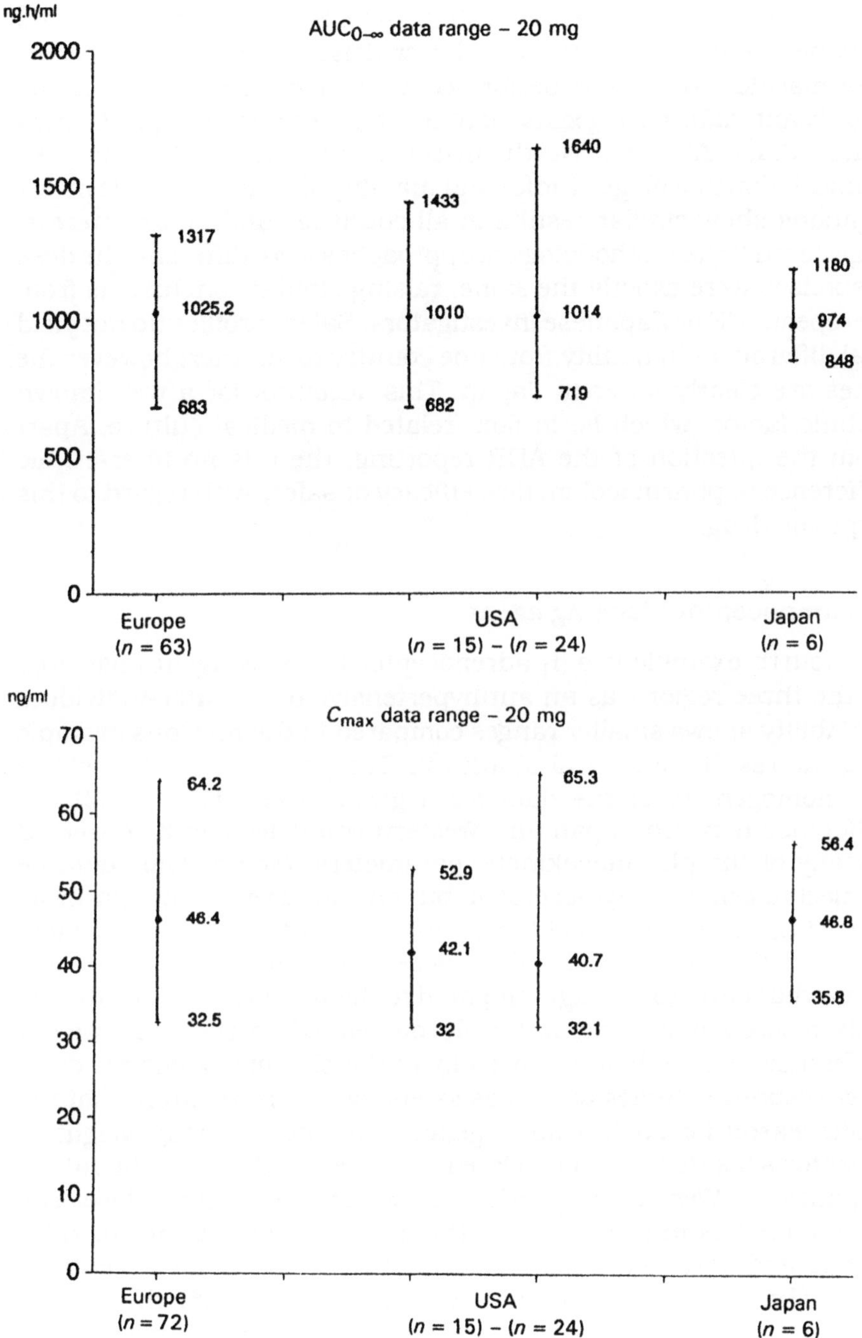

Figure 15.2 β blocking agent: C_{max} and AUC data ranges following administration of 20 mg

64 volunteers in Europe and 130 in the US, were compared to six Japanese subjects, which can be criticised. However, a specific pharmacokinetic study performed in Europe confirms that no significant difference exists between four ethnic groups (Caucasians, Black Africans, North African Arabs, South East Asians). Clinical pharmacology studies and mainly polysomnographic investigations show similar results in all countries and, more interestingly, even if the methodological approaches were different, the dose responses were exactly the same, raising similar conclusions from European, US or Japanese investigators. Safety profiles do not yield real differences in quality from one country to another; however the rates are clearly lower in Japan. This accounts for a well known "ethnic factor" which is, in fact, related to medical culture. Apart from the question of the ADR reporting, there is no inter-ethnic difference in pharmacokinetics, efficacy or safety with regard to this hypnotic drug.

β_1 adrenoceptor blocking agent

The fourth example is a β_1 adrenoceptor blocking agent registered in the three regions as an antihypertensive drug. Inter-individual variability shows smaller ranges compared to the previous example and the results of several studies in Europe and US demonstrate the homogeneity of the data for a given dose (Figure 15.2). No difference between Japan and Western countries can be observed for any of the pharmacokinetic parameters. Metabolism could be subject to genetic polymorphism, but only for a very minor pathway involving less than 10% of the catabolism, which can be neglected. However the recommended daily dose range registered in Japan is somewhat lower (5–20 mg) compared to the Western one (10–40 mg). This discrepancy could naturally be related to the body weight difference. In fact, looking carefully at the pharmacodynamic data, dose response studies as well as safety data, it is apparent that the main reason for such a not a genetic one (height/body weight or receptor sensitivity...), but related to medical culture as the rate of Japanese or Western responders is the same for a given dose. The difference lies in the choice of the acceptable incidence of side-effects and essentially the rate of "bradycardia". If the acceptable limit of bradycardia in one country is between 2 and 3%, the optimal dose and the rate of responders will be lower than in another country where the acceptable limit is 3–5%. In Europe, and even more so in the US, the practitioner is supposed to cure the patient, while in

Japan the practitioner's primary duty is not to harm his patient. In the case of this drug, the approved range of daily doses is lower in Japan and the expected rate of responders is consequently lower; in contrast, the safety is better when considering the effects related to β blockade. It can be concluded for this drug that there is an ethnic difference which does not involve genetic factors, but there is no difference in dose response.

α_1 adrenergic receptor antagonist

The last compound of this review is an α_1 adrenergic receptor antagonist developed in Europe and Japan. The pharmacokinetic parameters are subject to a large inter-individual variability in both areas. However, when plotting C_{max} and AUC individual values, the range of the Japanese data fits well into the range of the European data for three different doses. Upper and lower European limits are larger than the Japanese ones, but here again 65–99 Western subjects have to be compared to six Japanese subjects for the same dose. The intra-ethnic variability, estimated to be 50% or more, is larger than the inter-ethnic variability which is around 20–25%; all parameters show consistent values in both countries for absorption, metabolism and elimination. Pharmacodynamic studies demonstrate consistent results as well, even if sometimes the rating scales are not exactly the same. The Japanese safety profile is qualitatively similar to the European one for the same range of doses. However, the optimal dose proposed by the investigators from the dose finding studies in Japan was 25% lower than the European recommended daily dose in order to minimise the risk of haemodynamic effects. For this compound also, the apparent "ethnic difference" which is observed is linked to cultural differences rather than genetic polymorphism or drug response.

Conclusion

This brief retrospective review of five heterogeneous drug families found no pharmacogenetically linked differences between Caucasian and Japanese subjects. With regard to pharmacokinetic parameters, intra-ethnic variability was always higher than inter-ethnic variability. However, we encountered many discrepancies in the studies which were investigated. For instance, number of samples, sampling times, detection limits in HPLC are major factors for C_{max} determination and the calculation of AUC, T_{max}, $T\,\raisebox{0.4ex}{\scriptsize 1}/_2$, etc.

Differences in methods might contribute to the apparent variations of the values, which is also true for formulation characteristics and other factors such as study conditions, all of which prohibit statistical analysis of the data comparison. Body weight appeared to be a less influential factor than expected; the most striking differences were the number of subjects per study and the clinical trial methodology, particularly in Phase II and III. For these reasons, in order to make any conclusions in the field of drug response, it will be necessary to harmonise the methodology of drug development – principles and technical aspects – and in addition to the pharmacokinetic parameters, pharmacodynamics, efficacy and the safety profile will also have to be considered since "no kinetic difference" does not automatically imply "no difference in clinical response".

Acknowledgement

We would like to thank Ms Nathalie Robert and Ms Christiane Kaddour for their help in preparing this work.

16
Current status of CMR survey on inter-ethnic differences in clinical responsiveness

CHRISTINE HARVEY, NEIL McAUSLANE, CYNDY LUMLEY and STUART WALKER

Summary

1. The scientific basis for the limited acceptance of foreign clinical data by regulatory authorities when reviewing marketing applications for new medicines has yet to be determined. Detailed information on each phase of clinical development for 21 compounds studied in both Japanese and Western subjects has therefore been analysed to determine the clinical implications of any differences between regions in pharmacokinetic or clinical responsiveness.

2. The findings from initial analyses of kinetic information suggest that for the majority of compounds there were no inter-ethnic differences in absorption, pharmacokinetics or metabolism which had any basis on genotype. Differences in culture and medical practice have been highlighted between Japan and the West, which have contributed to the use of lower doses of some medicines and a lower reported incidence of adverse events in Japanese subjects.

3. No differences between the West and Japan in clinical effectiveness that were not due to methodological reasons have been found. However, it is important to address whether clinical trials, as currently conducted, are capable of identifying differences related to genetic polymorphisms.

Introduction

There is currently limited acceptance of foreign clinical data by regulatory authorities when reviewing marketing applications for new medicines. In some cases this is due to specific regulations, whilst in others, foreign clinical data is not widely accepted due to differences in medical practice. In Japan, for example, there is a requirement for pharmacokinetic studies, dose finding, and (Phase III) comparative clinical trials to be conducted in Japanese subjects, even though similar studies may have already been carried out in subjects of other ethnic origin (Anon, 1993). Recently, US regulations have been changed to allow for the use of non-US data as the sole basis for approval as long as certain conditions are met, for example, "foreign data should be applicable to US populations and US medical practice". Whilst it is accepted that companies may wish to conduct trials in local populations for marketing purposes, the scientific basis for repeating studies has yet to be determined. As the costs of drug development increase, and as companies become more international, there is greater awareness of this problem.

Of the three regions (Japan, USA, EC), Japan has the most genetically homogeneous population and the US has the most heterogeneous population. Ethnic genetic variation between the major ethnic divisions worldwide only accounts for approximately 11% of the total individual genetic variation. Inter-ethnic genetic variation, such as the varying ethnic frequency of genetic polymorphisms of the cytochrome P_{450} enzymes, is likely to have considerably less impact on drug kinetics and dynamics than other non-racial genetic factors or environmental influences. Any type of inter-individual variation in drug metabolism, whether ethnically linked or not, is most marked for drugs which display a narrow therapeutic window between effective and toxic dose. The genetic component of inter-individual variation in drug responsiveness is more easily characterised and quantified than that derived from environmental factors, including cultural factors, dietary and smoking habits, body size, and differences in medical practice, all of which may influence drug responsiveness.

The Japanese Ministry of Health and Welfare (MHW) has undertaken a study in Japan, looking at pharmacokinetic differences in Phase I studies for products covering a wide range of therapeutic classes, which have been approved in Japan since 1985. The results of this survey provide useful information on differences in Phase I pharmacokinetic parameters. However, it does not address differences in Phase II and III clinical responsiveness. The CMR has therefore initiated a survey in Europe and the USA to determine the clinical implications of any differences in pharmacokinetic or clinical responsiveness in Phase I, II or III studies.

Methodology

The objective of the CMR study is to collect data on compounds which have been clinically evaluated in Japanese and Western populations, in order to identify and characterise differences in clinical responsiveness. Compounds approved or submitted in Japan since 1985, which have been evaluated in both Japanese and Western subjects, are included. Following discussion and consultation with a number of experts, most notably the European Federation of Pharmaceutical Industries' Associations (EFPIA) expert working party for this International Conference on Harmonisation (ICH) topic, the Centre for Medicines Research (CMR) designed a detailed questionnaire covering all stages of clinical development and invited 14 US and 23 European companies to participate in this study. The data collected include approval information (dates of approvals, dosage and indications), detailed information on each phase of clinical development (healthy volunteers, Phase II dose response studies, major Phase III clinical trials), and adverse reactions associated with these trials for the three geographic areas (USA, Japan and Europe).

Results: preliminary analyses

Preliminary analyses on the first 21 compounds received have been undertaken. This cohort of 21 compounds comes from 12 companies (7 European and 5 American) and represents a range of therapeutic classes (Figure 16.1) and pharmacological modes of action. Seventeen of the compounds are either approved or an application has been submitted to the regulatory authorities. The remaining four compounds have undergone studies in Japan but are either still being developed or development has been terminated. The indications of use were similar in each region for all compounds except four, where, in Japan, there were additional indications.

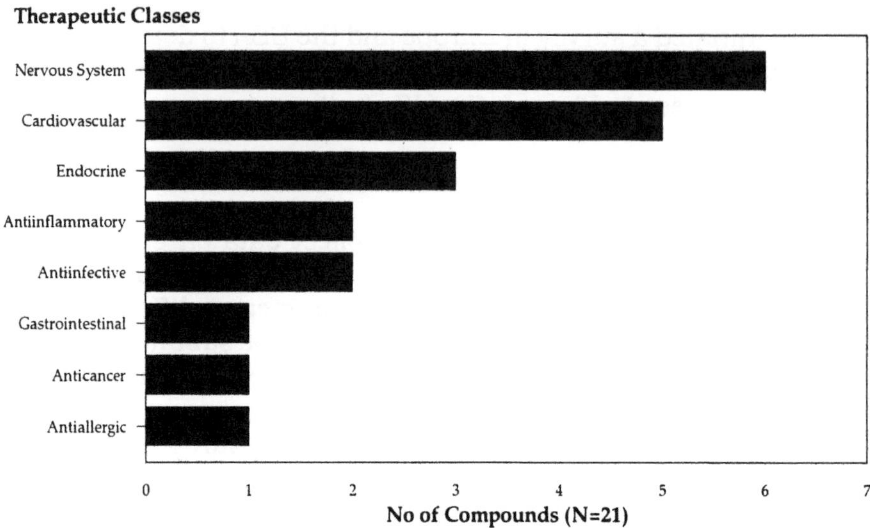

Figure 16.1 Therapeutic classes represented in the preliminary analysis on 21 compounds approved or submitted in the West and Japan

Differences in trial methodology

Numbers of subjects

There is anecdotal evidence to suggest that the numbers of subjects enrolled into clinical trials in Japan are lower than those included in corresponding trials conducted in Western countries. Respondents were asked to provide information on numbers of subjects in Phase I trials, in Phase II dose-finding studies, and in Phase III pivotal trials. Differences in indications make it difficult to compare numbers in trials for very different compounds, so data has been expressed as ratios for each compound (i.e. patients in Phase I trial Europe/patients in Phase I trial Japan, for the same compound). In all cases, single indications have been compared. The results are shown in Figure 16.2.

There appears to be extensive regional variation in the numbers of healthy volunteers included in Phase I studies, which is enhanced by the relatively small numbers of subjects tested. The average numbers of Phase I subjects for the three regions show considerable differences. Although no information was provided on the dates of Phase I studies, it is assumed that since the majority of these compounds were developed by Western companies, they were first tested in Western subjects, and Japanese trials probably occurred at a later date. The ratios for numbers of Phase II dose-finding trial

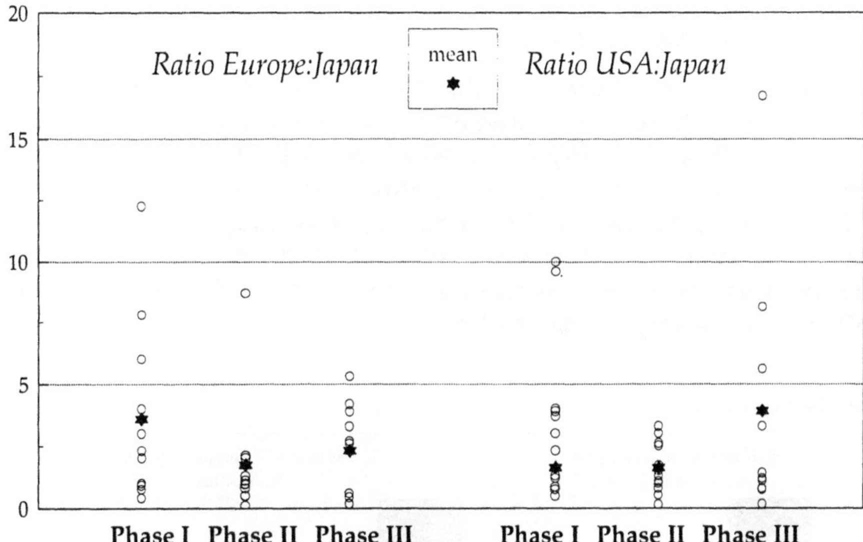

Figure 16.2 Individual compound and mean ratio of patients Europe/Japan and USA/Japan for Phase I, II, III clinical trials

subjects are lower, with the regions showing more similarity in numbers. More variation is observed for Phase III pivotal studies, and the numbers included in US pivotal trials are greater than those in European studies. Of the three areas, the lowest number of patients used in the evaluation of compounds was in Japan.

Phase II and III trial design

It is often suggested that data from Japanese clinical studies is derived largely from open trials, and is therefore not readily accepted by foreign regulators. Most respondents to this survey provided details of the design of Phase II dose-finding studies and of Phase III pivotal studies. From this preliminary analysis 15 compounds were tested in Phase II open dose-finding studies, with seven of these tested *only* in open studies in Japan. By comparison, 11 compounds were tested in open studies in the West, but only one of these was tested only in an open study. None of these compounds were tested in an open Phase III pivotal study in any of these regions. The majority of Phase III trials were randomised and double blind in design, but there were differences between the regions in the use of placebo and reference compounds.

Dosing and frequency of dosing

For each compound the respondents were asked if there were any inter-ethnic differences in dose and/or frequency of dosing in Phase III studies. In 4/21 compounds no answer was given but for ten of the remaining 17 compounds the company indicated that there were differences in dosing and/or frequency of dosing (Figure 16.3). In all cases medical practice was cited as the reason although for four compounds there were additional reasons, including commercial, efficacy and safety considerations.

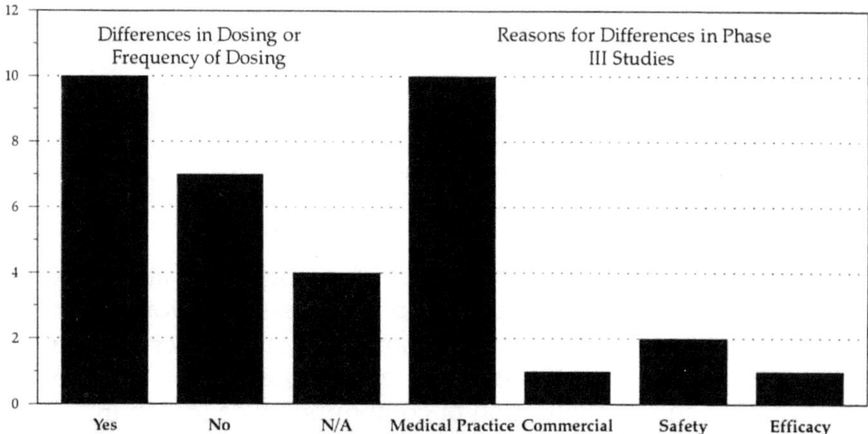

Figure 16.3 Number of compounds in which a difference in dosing or frequency of dosing was observed in Phase III studies between the West and Japan and the reasons for these differences

Inter-ethnic differences in Phase I studies

Although detailed information from Phase I studies has been collected, in this analysis only overall assessments of inter-ethnic differences in absorption, pharmacokinetics and metabolism and elimination have been considered. As shown below, the preliminary results indicate that differences have been seen in absorption, pharmacokinetic parameters, metabolism and elimination but these seem to be related mainly to methodology and study design differences between the three regions rather than any real inter-ethnic differences. In two cases there was a theoretical possibility for the metabolism to be influenced by genetic polymorphism but in neither case has a population subset been identified.

Absorption

If Phase I studies were conducted in more than one region for a compound, respondents were asked to indicate if there were any differences between regions in the absorption of the drug. In the case of 6/21 compounds no data was available and in four of these cases the compounds were administered intravenously. For 14 of the remaining 15 compounds, no differences in absorption were reported. A difference was reported with one compound, a cardiovascular (compound A, β-blocker), and the reason given is that different formulations were used. The non US formulation has been shown to be less bioavailable when compared to the US formulation.

Pharmacokinetic parameters

Each respondent was asked to indicate if they conducted studies in subjects from more than one region, whether there were any differences in pharmacokinetics. The parameters assessed included C_{max}, $T_{1/2}$, AUC_{0-24h}, volume of distribution and protein binding. Differences were reported for 4/21 compounds in this preliminary

Table 16.1 Pharmacokinetic differences

Therapeutic class	Reason for differences in pharmacokinetics	Clinical implications
A[*]. CVS (β-blocker)	Difference in bioavailability between US and non-US formulations	BP lowering effects may differ between formulations
B[*]. Antibacterial (Cephalosporin)	Differences in route of administration between Europe (drip infusion) and USA and Japan (i.v. bolus injection)	None
C[*]. Antiallergic (Antihistamine)	Difference in study design between Europe and Japan with T_{max} and $T_{1/2}$ being measured at different time points	None
D[*]. Hypnotic (Benzodiazepine)	Not known	None

[*] Compound identifier

analysis. The reasons for these differences and their clinical implications are shown in Table 16.1.

Metabolism/elimination

Three compounds were not metabolised to any extent and were excreted mostly unchanged. The remaining 18 compounds all undergo in the main Phase I and II type metabolism. All compounds/metabolites were excreted either by the renal and/or biliary routes. For only two of these 18 compounds were any of the known pathways of metabolism subject to genetic polymorphism (Table 16.2). In neither case were any differences seen between Western and Japanese healthy volunteers and there was no evidence of any population subsets.

Only one of the 17 compounds for which data was provided showed any differences between healthy volunteers in the three regions in metabolism/elimination of the drug or its active metabolites. This was a calcium antagonist (Compound F) which had quantitative differences in AUC of the metabolites. However, this difference was not believed by the company to be significant.

Differences in clinical effectiveness/response

For six compounds there was no data available on differences between the regions in clinical effectiveness/response. Of the remaining 15 compounds, only three showed such differences. As shown in Table 16.3, all differences in clinical effectiveness appear to be due to methodological differences between the three regions and the use of lower doses, rather than a real difference in how the patients were affected or responded to the drug.

Differences in adverse reactions

There was considerable inter-ethnic variation in adverse reactions during clinical trials with 9/17 compounds showing some regional difference. Typically, these differences were fewer types and lower frequencies in Japanese patients, though in all cases they had no significant implications for the development of the compound. Two respondents thought that lower Japanese doses were responsible for the reduced incidence of adverse reactions in Japanese trials. Explanations for inter-ethnic variation for the other seven compounds, where reactions were of a similar type but at a lower

Table 16.2 Compounds metabolised by pathways subject to genetic polymorphism

Therapeutic class	Metabolism
A[*]. CVS (β-blocker)	Undergoes aromatic ring oxidation, aliphatic side chain oxidation and glucuronidation
E[*]. Antidepressant	Metabolised by liver enzyme P_{450} system

[*] Compound identifier

Table 16.3 Reasons for differences in clinical effectiveness

Therapeutic Class	Reasons for Differences
F[*]. Cardiovascular (Ca^{2+} antagonist)	The differences seen were due to the use of lower doses in Japan. In Europe and USA the compound was evaluated on safety and efficacy compared to safety, efficacy and 'usefulness' in Japan. The Japanese emphasis on global/ subjective improvement rates favours the positive efficacy results seen with the lower dosage used in Japan
G[*]. Antiulcer (H_2 antagonist)	Differences seen were explained by the way in which clinical trials were evaluated in the West compared to Japan: blinding vs. none, use of placebo/comparators and grading system
H[*]: Cardiovascular	Blood pressure was measured at different times in the Western trials to that in the Japanese trials. This led to an apparent difference in dose/response. However when blood pressure was measured at the same time point no differences were seen in dose/response, so the difference was due to study design rather than any real inter-ethnic difference

[*] Compound identifier

Table 16.4 Explanations for inter-ethnic variations in adverse reactions

- cultural differences – use of preferred terms
- reporting differences
- differences in data collection
- differences in trial design and reporting
- different assessment methods
- Japan 'appears' to have a lower frequency
- drug 'seemed' better tolerated in Japan – reporting?

incidence, are shown in Table 16.4. For four compounds no details of adverse reactions were provided.

Overall there was no correlation between lower Japanese dosing levels and a lower incidence of adverse reactions in Japanese subjects. For the nine compounds in which differences in adverse reactions were observed, over half (five) were used at the same dose in Japan and the West, and the other four compounds were used at doses between two- and four-fold lower in Japanese patients. Likewise, of the compounds for which there were no differences in adverse reactions, approximately half (four) were used at the same dose in the West and Japan while four were used at a lower dose in Japan.

Benefit/risk assessment

For 17/21 compounds analysed to date, no differences in the overall benefit/risk assessment between the three regions have been evident. For the remaining four compounds, no information was given or such assessments have not yet been made.

Summary of CMR analyses

This paper describes preliminary analyses carried out on the first 21 compounds received by the CMR. The findings from initial analyses of kinetic information on drugs clinically developed in the West and in Japan suggest that for the majority of compounds there were no inter-ethnic differences in absorption, pharmacokinetics or metabolism which had any basis on genotype. Furthermore, none of the observed variations had any significance for the clinical development of these compounds. However, the results do highlight some of the differences in both culture and medical practice which exist, particularly between the West and Japan. Differences in medical practice contribute to the use of lower doses of some drugs in Japanese subjects and to the lower reported incidence of adverse reactions in these patients. There are also some differences in the design of trials, particularly for Phase II dose-finding studies, more of which are open trials in Japan, though the majority of Phase III pivotal studies from all areas were of double blind, controlled randomised design. American trials include more patients than corresponding trials for the same drugs in either Europe or Japan, and Japan evaluates drugs in fewer patients than the other regions.

Despite the wide range of therapeutic categories and metabolic pathways represented by this cohort of compounds, there were no differences between the regions in clinical effectiveness that were not due to methodological reasons between the three regions. No inter-ethnic differences in risk/benefit assessment were seen in these analyses. It should however be remembered that this analysis has been carried out on a small number of compounds and caution is required in drawing conclusions from such a small cohort. Although further information is being collected, it is apparent from the Workshop discussions that one of the main issues which needs to be addressed is whether clinical trials, as currently conducted, are capable of identifying differences related to genetic polymorphisms.

Reference

Anon (1993). In: *Drug Approval and Licensing Procedures in Japan 1992.* Yakugyo Jiho Co. Ltd, Tokyo.

SESSION III

THE RELEVANCE OF INTER-ETHNIC DIFFERENCES FOR DRUG DEVELOPMENT AND REGISTRATION

17
Implications for the design and interpretation of Phase III clinical trials

LUC BALANT, MARIANNE GEX-FABRY and
ANDRONIKI BALANT-GORGIA

Summary

1. This paper discusses some methodological aspects introduced by new approaches to the conduct of Phase IIb and Phase III clinical trials in the context of inter-ethnic differences in drug behaviour, tolerance and response.

2. If a new chemical entity is intended to be used in different ethnic settings, the implementation of population approaches such as the pharmacokinetic screen or population kinetic models might be a cost-effective means of detecting inter-ethnic differences in drug effects.

3. Randomised concentration-controlled or concentration-monitored clinical trials can be adapted to the problems raised by new drug development in different ethnic groups. Although the implementation of the former may be premature, most of the elements necessary to perform the latter are current practice.

4. In addition to data analysis strategies, many unresolved issues remain to be clarified if large scale clinical trials are to be performed in multi-ethnic settings. These relate to pharmaco-geography, protocols and research instruments, biological data and regulatory aspects. However, common sense and scientific ethics will be more important than strict adherence to guidelines.

Introduction

In 1982, Kalow introduced his review on "Ethnic differences in drug metabolism" stating that: *"...the literature contains a number of examples of differences between populations in drug metabolizing capacity. Although this topic has been discussed previously as part of pharmacogenetics review, it deserves a new effort with different emphasis on a recently expanded data base. The topic should help improve understanding of human biology, and is of practical significance in pharmacology and toxicology"*. Ten years later the same statement is still true and considerable knowledge has been acquired at the molecular biology level. As a matter of fact, a recently published book on pharmacogenetics (Kalow, 1992) contains important and extensive information on inter-ethnic differences in drug metabolism. Simultaneously, it has become evident that different ethnic groups may also show differences in response to the administration of drugs. However, the implications for drug development, licensing and registration in the context of the new "4 W" environment (i.e. What and Why to present for World Wide drug registration) are still largely unknown. In parallel to these developments, pharmacokinetic/pharmacodynamic (PK/PD) relationships are becoming of importance, as exemplified by a recent conference (Peck *et al.*, 1992). This paper concentrates on some methodological aspects introduced by these new approaches to the conduct of Phase IIb and Phase III clinical trials in the context of inter-ethnic differences in drug behaviour, tolerance and response.

Goal and scope of clinical trials

The potential problems raised by finding *"dose–concentration–effect–response"* relationships in the context of inter-ethnic differences have been discussed in detail in a recent paper (Balant and Bechtel, 1994) which also contains definitions related to the terminology used herein. In particular, studies performed in patients in order to explore such relationships have been termed for the present purpose "Phase IIa" studies, and the term "Phase IIb" clinical trials will be used to indicate that these investigations are direct precursors of the large scale Phase III clinical trials. As a consequence, it is implied that Phase IIa investigations still bear many features of clinical pharmacological studies performed in healthy volunteers, whereas Phase IIb studies are methodologically closer to Phase III clinical trials.

Phase IIb studies

The principal goal of Phase IIb studies is to provide unequivocal evidence of the desired therapeutic effect. A second major goal is to gain information that will guide Phase III clinical trials. Often, however, Phase II is shortened and hence, the extra time needed to explore the full dose range and various dose intervals to obtain good dose– and concentration–response information may not be committed. Undoubtedly, this approach can be successful and it can be rapid, but on too many occasions failure to define dose–concentration–response relationships leads to unacceptable toxicity or adverse effects, marginal evidence of effectiveness and lack of information on how to individualise dosing. This is especially true when Phase III is designed with a series of concurrent studies that allow no opportunity for the results of one trial to influence the design of subsequent studies. It is in this context that the concept of *randomised concentration-controlled or concentration monitored clinical trials* has been proposed (Peck, 1992). In this type of study, subjects are either randomised into separate ranges of average plasma drug concentrations achieved by PK-controlled dosage, or blood samples are taken and patients are categorised *a posteriori* as a function of the measured blood concentrations of the active principle. As discussed below, these concepts can certainly be adapted to the particular problems raised by new drug development in different ethnic groups, independently of the choice to conduct such studies simultaneously or sequentially in different ethnic settings.

Phase III clinical studies

For reasons already discussed (Balant and Bechtel, 1994), systemic drug concentration data during Phase III clinical trials should ideally be routinely obtained on a survey basis to help explain unusual responses, to suggest the possibility for either the presence or lack of drug–drug and drug–disease interactions, and to identify other unanticipated variability such as metabolic heterogeneity (Balant *et al.*, 1989) or potential inter-ethnic differences. This is particularly important in the context of a worldwide development of a new chemical entity taking place in a multi-ethnic environment since even a well-developed and carefully planned programme cannot anticipate all possibilities. Moreover, specific studies of all possible subsets of patients and all potential interactions are costly, time consuming, and probably unnecessary. Accordingly, as discussed below, new approaches allowing the extraction of more information from available data must be implemented. As an example, the *pharmacokinetic screen* (a small number of blood level measurements taken in some or all patients), coupled with integrated analyses of effectiveness and safety data, or more *formal population models,* can be used to identify and quantify important demographic and other subset differences. The more complex approach using "population models" is based on a more intensive data collection scheme, more elaborate PK/PD models and a higher level of sophistication of the statistical methodology than the pharmacokinetic screen (Aarons, 1991; Vozeh, 1992; Ebelin *et al.,* 1992). These concepts have recently been discussed, and controversial positions have been expressed. It is not the intention of the authors to discuss the advantages or disadvantages of this approach in the development of a new drug under normal conditions. However, it seems interesting to discuss whether these concepts should be considered and possibly adapted to the requirements of drug development in different ethnic groups.

Methods for identification of variability during Phase III clinical trials

Introducing variability: impact on study design

Large scale Phase III clinical trials are usually designed to have maximum efficiency for rejecting the null hypothesis of no treatment effect, the usual design being the *randomised controlled clinical trial.* As such, these studies are usually one factor (drug), two-level (zero dose, and maximum safe dose) designs which measure a single univariate endpoint per patient (e.g. time to a clinical event or occurrence or not of some predefined endpoint). They are generally applied to a homogeneous patient population in order to reduce variability in patients and increase the power of statistical tests. When overall efficacy of standard treatments is the central question, such designs serve well. However, the central issue of ultimate efficacy for modern drugs concerns maximising the benefit/risk ratio for individual patients (Sheiner, 1992). These "individuals" may stem from apparently homogeneous populations or from populations where racial and/or environmental factors may play a decisive role in drug efficacy and toxicity. In this context, a series of questions must be answered: what is the relationship between input profile and dose magnitude on the one hand, and beneficial or harmful pharmacological effects, on the other? How does this relationship vary with individual patient characteristics? Studies designed to answer these questions must be multi-factorial (i.e. study several treatments simultaneously) and multi-level (e.g. study multiple dose magnitudes). They must also measure multiple (over time), possibly multi-variate responses in a deliberately heterogeneous patient population (Sheiner, 1992). Heterogeneity may be introduced by age, gender, co-medications, concurrent diseases or racial and life habit diversities. In order to improve the discriminatory power of data analysis, it is probably valuable to obtain some type of information on dose–concentration relationships and, accordingly, it follows logically that it may be of interest to systematically take some blood samples from the patients enrolled in Phase III clinical trials. This information is crucial for the separation of pharmacokinetic from pharmacodynamic sources of variability (Balant and Bechtel, 1994).

Population approaches

Clearly, measurement of drug concentrations during Phase IIb and III clinical trials requires pharmacokinetic and statistical methods which are different from those used in traditional formal pharmacokinetic studies in which many data points are available in few subjects. In the broadest sense, the term *"population approach"* (as used in the context of pharmacokinetics) applies to any method used to study the variability of drug/metabolite concentrations in blood or plasma and the causes of this variability (i.e. co-variables), as well as sources of variability arising from pharmacodynamic factors. This variability is due to the patients' characteristics such as genetic background, age, gender, weight or associated diseases (i.e. intrinsic co-variables) or to factors such as co-medication, nutritional habits or other environmental conditions (i.e. extrinsic co-variables). Population approaches imply that both sources of variability are investigated and quantified. This means that the potential influence of individual co-variables must be looked for and that the magnitude of this influence must be estimated. In addition, the "unexplained" variability is also estimated. The method implies the investigation of causes of variability in the general population in order to detect subpopulations at risk of showing abnormal kinetic or dynamic behaviours with the aim to finally identify those individuals or specific subpopulations for which special dosage adjustments are needed. It is thus crucial to understand that in spite of the name given to these approaches, "population methods" are basically aimed to fulfil the needs of individual patients.

Pharmacokinetic screen

The term "pharmacokinetic screen" has been proposed by Temple in 1983 and 1985 to describe a blood sampling method and a strategy of data analysis performed during large-scale Phase III clinical trials. The concept was initially proposed specifically for the study of pharmacokinetic variability induced by ageing, but it can clearly be extended to other sources of variability. The rationale of this approach is that because of logistic and ethical reasons, it is improbable that traditional pharmacokinetic experimentation can be carried out on each and every patient subpopulation. It is thus possible, at best, to hope for one or two blood samples per patient being obtained during clinical trials. In this proposal, collection of trough levels is recommended to detect patient groups at risk of an altered dose–concentration–effect relationship. Data interpretation based on data collected according to this pharmacokinetic screen concept can provide valuable information on the factors susceptible to alter dose–concentration relationships, but it must be realised that the "one-point-per-patient" sampling scheme may not necessarily lead to the full characterisation of pharmacokinetic parameters of the drug in specific subpopulations. The pharmacokinetic screen is an observational rather than experimental study. Strengths of such an approach include simplicity in terms of data collection and statistical analysis, representativeness of the patient population and early detection of atypical behaviour of the drug in some patients or groups of patients. Weaknesses include, as already stated, limited pharmacokinetic information and the need for a relatively large number of data to detect significant factors.

Population pharmacokinetics

A more complex approach, termed population pharmacokinetics (Aarons, 1991), is based on a more intensive data collection scheme (Vozeh, 1992; Ebelin *et al.*, 1992). Several drug levels (e.g. two to four) are needed from a majority of patients, at different times relative to the last dose. Its main advantage is to be able to describe the full pharmacokinetic profile and to allow estimation of relevant population parameters. Its drawback is the need for more complex "PK-population models" and increased sophistication of the required statistical techniques and software. In summary, any approach in which a pharmacokinetic model is used to estimate mean kinetic characteristics of a drug and their variance, as well as the influence of co-variables, can be termed population kinetics independently of study design, data analysis strategy and computer software. This distinction between integrated kinetic/statistical model specification and software implementation is important since, unfortunately for the clarity of the issue, the computer package NONMEM, developed in a pioneering way by Sheiner and Beal in San Francisco in the late 1970s (Beal and Sheiner, 1980) has (in the understanding of many) become synonymous with population pharmacokinetics. This is, in part, because it is an easily available and widely used software package and, in part, because the name of this software is the abbreviation for the statistical approach to population kinetics implemented in the program (i.e. the Nonlinear Mixed Effect Model). Finally, it must be stated that despite the fact that most of the available literature on population approaches concerns kinetics, these methods can also be successfully applied for the study of drug effects.

PK/PD integration and inter-ethnic differences in drug behaviour and action

It is clear that the potential of an integrated PK/PD approach depends on the interplay between pharmacokinetic and metabolic profiles, pharmacological activity, therapeutic margin, clinical endpoints, indications and patient populations or subpopulations. Similar considerations certainly apply for the use of this approach in the context of the transfer of a medication from one racial group to another. It is clear that an understanding of the behaviour of the drug in different ethnic groups is then of crucial importance. Indeed, during new drug development, the pharmaceutical industry can be expected to devote time and resources to investigate the potential impact of inter-ethnic differences in drug metabolism and response for an active substance for which it can be assumed from preclinical or clinical data that such differences might be clinically relevant. It is, however, not practical to ask industry to perform, systematically, wide scale clinical trials in a full range of different ethnic settings for all new chemical entities intended for human use. Costs and timing would become prohibitive. In view of these limitations, there might be a case to utilise *ad hoc* population approaches during Phase IIb and III clinical trials in order to gain some insight into potential inter-ethnic differences in drug fate and effects.

Impact of variability assessment on study design and clinical data interpretation

Use of pharmacokinetic information

Discrepancy between theory and practice?

As discussed previously, there is a general tendency to use strict inclusion and exclusion criteria for Phase IIb and III studies in order to maximise the chances of reaching statistically significant results in favour of the drug under development. This leads, however, to "information-poor" data as far as different co-variables such as age, race, cultural aspects or concomitant diseases are concerned. It is thus necessary to reconsider this attitude if a new chemical entity is intended to be used in different ethnic settings and, as discussed above, implementation of population approaches such as the *pharmacokinetic screen* or the more complex *population kinetic models* might be cost-effective means of detecting inter-ethnic differences in drug effects.

If it can be accepted that there are potential advantages to measure blood concentrations of drug and active metabolites during Phase IIb and III clinical trials and that the conceptual framework for the interpretation of such data sets exists, then the question which must be answered is, as stated by Sheiner and Benet in 1985: *"Why is this approach often viewed with some reluctance within the pharmaceutical industry and why is it only exceptionally used in the context of new drug development despite the fact that it has been advocated for about 10 years?"* (Balant, 1985, 1993). Possible answers may be found in practical issues which remain to be solved before such measurements and, consequently, population approaches can be fully implemented as complements to the methods traditionally used in new drug development. One point of misunderstanding which must immediately be clarified is the fact that a drug development programme based on clinical trials during which blood levels have been measured in no way implies that routine drug monitoring will be necessary once the new drug reaches the market.

Specific study designs for blood sampling

In previous paragraphs, the ideas leading to the proposal of "concentration-controlled" or "monitored" clinical trials have briefly been mentioned. From its design it appears that the *randomised concentration-controlled clinical trial* is particularly useful in Phase IIa, and eventually IIb, for the characterisation of the dose–concentration–

effect relationships of a new active principle. However, its implementation in the frame of large scale multi-centre clinical trials is premature in view of the numerous issues which remain to be solved both from practical and statistical points of view. On the contrary, most of the elements necessary to perform *randomised concentration-monitored clinical trials* are today current practice, even if not performed on a routine basis. As previously discussed, study design is basically identical to the traditional way of performing clinical studies. Blood samples for drug concentration measurement can be obtained. Perhaps the only area where more work is needed is data analysis of clinical data and of drug concentration data when this additional information is available. These two aspects will be briefly discussed in the following paragraphs.

Logistical issues

Blood concentration measurements of the active principle are usually not performed during Phase III multi-centre clinical trials, and one objection often made is that this kind of pharmacokinetic data are "soft" due to poor control of drug administration, sampling time, sample handling and storage, analytical error and/or patient compliance. This is certainly a matter of concern and no population software will ever be able to magically transform the "garbage in, garbage out" problem into "lead in, gold out" alchemy. In any case, such variability factors will increase the "unexplained" variability which may result in concealing clinically relevant co-variables. It is evident that the rules of good clinical practice are a first step in increasing the quality of such data. Further improvement is certainly possible. Among the possible solutions one may propose concepts developed for the measurement of clinical biology and biochemistry data during large scale clinical trials. As an example, it is now accepted to entrust to specialised contract research organisations (CROs) for handling, shipping and analysing samples. Similar solutions are certainly adaptable to the centralised handling and measurement of drug concentrations, and some CROs and central laboratories are already performing such tasks with success.

Sparse kinetic data analysis

The concept of "sparse data" or "data-poor" studies relates to the number of drug concentrations available per individual patient. Normally, this low number is compensated for by the fact that numerous subjects (i.e. more than 100) are included in the analysis. Different strategies of data analysis have been proposed. For example, it is possible to combine into an explicit mathematical model both pharmacokinetic and statistical features, in order to describe variability and to detect the influential factors or clinically relevant co-variables. This is an integrated or "one-stage" approach of which the nonlinear mixed effects model proposed by Beal and Sheiner (1980) is a good and classical example, implemented in a widely used software (NONMEM). Other integrated approaches or "one-stage" methods have been proposed, but they are not yet generally available as software to be used by a large public. They include data analysis strategies based on the nonparametric maximum likelihood method (Mallet, 1986), Bayesian methods (Racine-Poon and Smith, 1990) and variants of the nonlinear mixed effect model (Amisaki and Tatsuhara, 1988; Lindstrom and Bates, 1990). The analysis of sparse data according to these methods certainly requires sophisticated methodologies and their complexity has led a number of people to shy away from them. The way forward is probably through co-operation between traditional pharmacokineticists and individuals who have the necessary skills in analysing sparse data. This is a crucial issue for the implementation of drug concentration measurements during Phase IIb and III clinical trials. It can also be proposed to use less sophisticated or "two-stage" approaches in which individual pharmacokinetic parameters are first estimated using a structural pharmacokinetic model and then related to demographic data using classical statistical methods such as univariate or multi-variate analyses, clustering and others. Such methods have been applied with success both to studies generating "data-rich" information (cyclosporine in 187 patients: Lindholm *et al.*, 1992) and "data-poor" kinetic results (isradipine in 252 patients: Laplanche *et al.*, 1991; clomipramine in 150 patients: Gex-Fabry *et al.*, 1990).

Strategies for clinical data analysis

One concern of clinicians and statisticians working in the pharmaceutical industry is the impact of the knowledge of active principle concentrations on clinical data analysis in the context of the well established "ended cohort" and "intent to treat" statistical methods. Among the questions usually raised, one can, for example, mention the problem linked to the ultimate classification of patients with undetectable drug concentrations in the active group or patients with abnormally high concentrations. It is clear that exclusion of patient subgroups based on drug concentrations can modify the apparent outcome of the study. This issue must be addressed by scientists in academia, the pharmaceutical industry and regulatory authorities if concentration measurement during clinical trials is to gain acceptance by those working in clinical departments within the industry.

Statistical significance and clinical relevance

As in any other situation encountered in drug development, data analysis can detect statistically significant differences in pharmacokinetic or pharmacodynamic characteristics which have no clinical relevance, as well as dismiss clinically important differences because they do not "show up" with statistical tests. Two complementary issues can be explored in this context. On the one hand, it is scientifically important to define (as well as possible) the means and variances of pharmacokinetic characteristics in a patient population, and to detect potentially influential co-variables using appropriate study designs and data analysis strategies. On the other hand, only deviations from a "normal" behaviour which have clinical relevance are ultimately important in the context of drug development, labelling and use. Clinical relevance necessarily includes consideration of therapeutic margin of the new drug, intended indications, as well as main target populations. Clinically relevant deviations will, necessarily, lead to warnings in the labelling, to contra-indications or to recommendations of altered dosage regimens. This implies that "deviations from normality" that are to be detected are generally of relatively important magnitude, and that data analysis strategies can be tailored in order to detect only those differences which are clinically relevant.

Practical problems raised by multi-ethnic Phase III clinical trials

Many questions can be raised in the context of planning and execution of multicentre clinical trials in multi-ethnic settings. In the following paragraphs only some of these issues will be briefly presented and discussed.

"Pharmaco-geography"

The decision to conduct clinical trials in a given geographic zone depends not only on the ethnic groups which are to be investigated

Table 17.1 Factors affecting the choice of location of clinical trials

The company:	Local company facilities; training in clinical research of local staff; logistical issues.
Investigators and patients:	Clinical research infrastructure; investigators' expertise; patients' availability; cultural realities (diagnoses, usual treatments...).
Country dependent realities:	Regulatory conditions; market size.

but also on numerous other factors such as those shown in Table 17.1.

All these components must be analysed in order to take a decision about the "best" locations to conduct multi-ethnic clinical trials and, consequently, such decisions are generally the result of a series of compromises. It must thus be accepted that the additional effort undertaken in order to explore inter-ethnic differences in drug behaviour and action are often obtained at the expenses of lower study design quality and execution as compared to "state of the art" clinical trials performed in highly sophisticated medical centres located in developed countries or urban areas of poorer countries.

Protocols and research instruments

The translation of a study protocol presents no major difficulties as such. However, the situation is more complicated if specific aspects are to be translated not only for language, but also from cultural points of views. The following examples may serve as illustrations of the numerous potential problems encountered in this respect.

In-patients versus out-patients: Depending on local conditions, the severity of a given disease may be quite different for in- or out-patients. Since this overall classification is often used to indicate severity, it is crucial to use more precise criteria.

Diagnostic criteria: Despite the year-long efforts of WHO to define diagnostic criteria that would be "universally" applicable, it must be realised that this a very difficult goal to achieve, in particular for diseases for which the cultural component is important. Depression is a good example of this type of disease and adequate provisions must then be implemented to ensure that patients are comparable in the different study locations.

Rating scales: Here again, it is not difficult to literally translate rating instruments from one language into another. However, it is much more difficult to ascertain that the meaning and the rating levels include the same conceptual bases in the two cultures. On occasions, this can even be observed for the translation of psychiatric rating scales from "American-English" to "Swiss-French" (Personal observations).

Clinical research forms (CRFs): The clinical research forms should, on the one hand, be written in all the native languages of the persons responsible for collecting the clinical data and, on the other hand, allow unambiguous data input in centralised data banks. This can theoretically be achieved by different methods such as multi-language CRFs, mono-language CRFs and data transcription. All methods have advantages and inconveniences, but the problems can usually be solved using modern data handling approaches. However, this necessitates within the company the presence of skilled personnel and the potential to work in the different languages used for the clinical trial under consideration. It is evident that such constraints are expensive.

Biological data

If clinical biochemistry and biology data are to be compared, it is important that they be "*a priori*" comparable. The following examples illustrate some of the potential difficulties in multi-ethnic settings when laboratory equipment is not necessarily identical.

Blood counts: This represents a minor problem as far as measurement techniques are considered. Some problems may be encountered as far as normal values are concerned in specific areas such as populations living at high altitudes, but this is probably more an academic question than a real problem.

Biochemistry: Clinical biochemistry tests from different laboratories are often performed using different methods. As a result, values are often given in different units with different "normal" ranges. The first problem can easily be overcome using *ad hoc* algorithms during data handling, but the second problem is much more difficult to control. This is made even more difficult if patients recruited in a study have different biological parameter values at inclusion in the study as compared to local reference populations. This is an area which certainly needs more attention before multi-ethnic trial methodologies can be fully validated. One potential solution is the use of "central clinical biology and biochemistry laboratories". However, for this centralised concept to be operational, blood and urine samples must arrive in good condition at the laboratory. This often means a tremendous pressure on time delays between sampling and analysis. Time reduction can be achieved under certain conditions, but logistics is a factor that should not be underestimated and it must be accepted that if the central laboratory is too far away from the sampling sites, other solutions must be envisaged. Among those solutions one may think of equipment and on the spot training of personnel to perform these determinations. Here again, cost might become prohibitive.

Regulatory aspects

Besides technical aspects, it is also important to consider some regulatory problems which may arise in the context of multi-ethnic clinical trials. There are no general recommendations that can be made to find solutions and they must be solved on a case by case basis.

Ethical committees

It is obligatory, according to the rules of good clinical practice, to have the approval of a recognised ethical committee before starting a clinical trial. However, in many countries such committees do not exist and alternative solutions must be sought.

Drug product

Importing a drug product for clinical trials may be difficult in some countries and it is sometimes problematic to store drugs in adequate facilities.

Archives for CRFs and final reports

Final reports and CRFs should be kept in a central site. However, it is sometimes mandatory to store this material in the country in which the clinical trial was performed. In addition, if the final report was written in a language different from the one in use in the country of the pharmaceutical company, it must be decided if a translation might be accepted as the "original" final report.

Conclusions

From a conceptual point of view it seems evident that there are some areas in new drug development in which the approach of sparse data analysis using drug concentration data obtained during medium to large scale clinical trials provides advantages over more traditional strategies (Balant *et al.*, 1990). Areas of particular interest include the detection of clinically important kinetic drug–drug interactions, genetic metabolic deficiencies, pharmacokinetic studies in neonates or elderly patients (Balant *et al.*, 1989). Interest for the measurement of drug concentrations during clinical trials has been expressed by regulatory agencies both in the USA (Peck, 1992) and Europe (Gundert-Remy, 1992), but it is generally recognised that work remains to be done before such approaches can be fully implemented in new drug development programmes. The authors are aware that many pharmaceutical companies have either the intention to test such methods or have already tested them. With a few exceptions this experience has not been made available to the scientific community by publication in scientific journals and it is consequently difficult to estimate the amount of experience already available in this field. It can, however, be argued that these studies were in general performed after the drug reached the market, and it is thus very important that the validity of the concept of drug concentration measurement during clinical trials be tested in real life conditions. This is the reason why a European Coordinated Action has been launched in the frame of COST B1 in order to explore the applicability of these concepts during new drug development.

However, in addition to data analysis strategies, many unsolved issues remain to be clarified if large scale clinical trials are to be performed in multi-ethnic settings. As in many other instances related to new drug development, common sense and scientific ethics will be more important than strict adherence to guidelines. It is thus mandatory to associate scientists from academia, the pharmaceutical industry and regulatory bodies in order to develop new strategies for the conduct of clinical trials in the context of worldwide development of new drugs.

References

Aarons L (1991). Population pharmacokinetics: Theory and practice. *Br J Clin Pharmacol*, **32**:669–670.

Amisaki T and Tatsuhara T (1988). An alternative two stage method via the EM-algorithm for the estimation of population pharmacokinetic parameters. *J Pharmacobio-Dyn*, **11**:335–348.

Balant LP (1985). Dosage des médicaments au cours des essais de phase III et de phase IV. *Méd Hyg,* **43**:2470–2473.

Balant LP (1993). Blood concentrations measurement in clinical trials. *Appl Clin Trials,* **2**:44–93.

Balant LP and Bechtel P (1994). Inter-ethnic differences in dose response studies. In: Walker SR, Lumley CE and McAuslane JAN (eds) *The Relevance of Ethnic Factors in the Clinical Evaluation of Medicines*. Kluwer Academic Publishers, Lancaster, pp. 27–48

Balant LP, Gundert-Remy U, Boobis AR and von Bahr Ch (1989). Relevance of genetic polymorphism in drug metabolism in the development of new drugs. *Eur J Clin Pharmacol,* **36**:551–554.

Balant LP, Roseboom H and Gundert-Remy U (1990). Pharmacokinetic criteria for drug research and development. In: Testa B (ed.) *Advances in Drug Research*. Academic Press, London, pp. 1–139.

Beal SL and Sheiner LB (1980). The NONMEM system. *Am Stat,* **34**:118–119.

Ebelin ME, Steimer JL, Laplanche R and Niederberger W (1992). An evaluation of population pharmacokinetics during drug development: Experiences with graphical exploratory analysis for isradipine and tropisetron. In: Rowland M and Aarons L (eds) *New Strategies in Drug Development and Clinical Evaluation: The Population Approach*. Commission of the European Communities (Coordinated Action COST B1), Luxembourg, pp. 131–141.

Gex-Fabry M, Balant-Gorgia AE, Balant LP and Garrone G (1990). Clomipramine metabolism: Model based analysis of variability factors from drug monitoring data. *Clin Pharmacokin,* **19**:241–255.

Gundert-Remy U (1992). Population approach in pharmacokinetics and pharmacodynamics – Views within regulatory agencies: Europe. In: Rowland M and Aarons L (eds) *New Strategies in Drug Development and Clinical Evaluation: The Population Approach*. Commission of the European Communities (Coordinated Action COST B1), Luxembourg, pp. 153–156.

Kalow W (1982). Ethnic differences in drug metabolism. *Clin Pharmacokin,* **7**:373–400.

Kalow W (1992). Pharmacoanthropology and the genetics of drug metabolism. In: Kalow W (ed.) *Pharmacogenetics of Drug Metabolism*. Pergamon Press, New York, pp. 865–877.

Laplanche R, Fertil B, Nüesch E, Jais JP, Niederberger W and Steimer JL (1991). Exploratory analysis of population pharmacokinetic data from clinical trials with application to isradipine. *Clin Pharmacol Ther,* **50**:39–54.

Lindholm A, Welsch M, Alton C and Kahan BD (1992). Demographic factors influencing cyclosporine pharmacokinetic parameters in patients with uremia: Racial differences in bioavailability. *Clin Pharmacol Ther*, **52**, 359–371.

Lindstrom MJ and Bates DM (1990). Nonlinear mixed effects models for repeated measures data. *Biometrics*, **46**:673–687.

Mallet A (1986) A maximum likelihood estimation method for random coefficient regression models. *Biometrika*, **73**:645–656.

Mallet A, Mentré F, Steimer JL and Lokiec F (1988). Nonparametric maximum likelihood estimation for population pharmacokinetics, with application to cyclosporine. *J Pharmacokin Biopharm*, **16**:311–327.

Peck CC (1992). Population approach in pharmacokinetics and pharmacodynamics: FDA view. In: Rowland M and Aarons L (eds) *New Strategies in Drug Development and Clinical Evaluation: The Population Approach.* Commission of the European Communities (Coordinated Action COST B1), Luxembourg, pp. 157–168.

Peck CC and co-authors (1992). Opportunities for integration of pharmacokinetics, pharmacodynamics, and toxicokinetics in rational drug development. *Clin Pharmacol Ther*, **51**:465–473.

Racine-Poon A and Smith AFM (1990). Population models. In: Berry DA (ed.), *Statistical Methodology in the Pharmaceutical Sciences*. Marcel Dekker, New York, pp. 139–162.

Sheiner LB (1992). Population approach in drug development: Rationale and basic concepts. In: Rowland M and Aarons L (eds) *New Strategies in Drug Development and Clinical Evaluation: The Population Approach.* Commission of the European Communities (Coordinated Action COST B1), Luxembourg, pp. 13–27.

Sheiner LB, Benet LZ (1985). Premarketing observational studies of population pharmacokinetics of new drugs. *Clin Pharmacol Ther*, **38**:481–487.

Temple R (1983). Discussion paper on the testing of drugs in the elderly, Washington, DC: Memorandum of the Food and Drug Administration of DHHS.

Temple R (1985). Food and Drug Administration's guidelines for clinical testing of drugs in the elderly. *Drug Information J*, **19**:483–486.

Vozeh S (1992). Applications of population approach to clinical pharmacokinetics and validation of results. In: Rowland M and Aarons L (eds) *New Strategies in Drug Development and Clinical Evaluation: The Population Approach*. Commission of the European Communities (Coordinated Action COST B1), Luxembourg, pp. 107–120.

18
Dose–utility relationships in diverse populations: ethnic, age, gender and cultural factors in efficacy and safety

LEIGH THOMPSON

Summary

1. Traditional clinical trials conducted in homogeneous populations have minimised variance so that the results define efficacy under the most optimal conditions. It is questionable whether these results can be extrapolated to the usual treatment of diverse populations, as many variables influence safety and efficacy.

2. It is important that clinical trial protocols, especially Phase III and IV, resemble to the fullest possible extent the use of the product expected in the world marketplace. Lilly has therefore revised its clinical trial strategies to assess multicultural dose–response effects in large scale global clinical trials.

3. The examples of substantial differences in efficacy and adverse events among patients of different ethnic origin suggest that estimations of efficiency in general use are best made from large global trials that admit widely diverse patients, with the results analysed by many defined factors.

Traditional clinical trial designs

Traditional clinical trials have minimised variance, maximised differences between means, and enhanced the power to show *statistically significant* differences between means by:

- restricting enrolment to relatively young healthy adults, predominantly males, who eschew unhealthy habits, comply with therapies, use few medications, and have few concomitant illnesses;
- choosing subjects and patients of average size and shape; and
- choosing excellent investigators with proven success in clinical trials who select optimum patients expected to comply with, and respond favourably to, the test medicine.

In such trials the drug kinetics and dynamics vary little. Small lot to lot or formulation to formulation differences might be found to be *statistically significant* even when in clinical practice these differences would be overwhelmed by the diversity of physicians, patients and practices.

In safety and efficacy trials with these designs, the results may define *"efficacy"* under the most optimal conditions, but can one extrapolate the results to the usual treatment of diverse populations? *"Effectiveness"* may await market experiences, which are always uncontrolled and haphazard trials.

Variables that influence drug safety and efficacy

If one is cautious in extrapolating the results of trials in primates to humans, why is there not equivalent concern in extrapolating results from a homogeneous population of young, thin, adult European male athletes to an elderly, ill, fat, diabetic Serbian woman or a tiny, starving Somali infant? In clinical trials, what has been seen of the outliers in distributions of kinetics, efficacy, or safety? Has the focus been on the mean or median? Is only the variance or standard error sufficient as a measure of dispersion? Is the distribution skewed or multimodal? Is there a cluster of unusual patients?

Drug kinetics, efficacy, and safety may be influenced by:

- correct patient diagnoses and the stage and severity of diseases;

- patient perceptions of the illness, investigator, therapies, and the protocol;
- patient cultural and personal tendencies to experience, remember, and report good and bad occurrences;
- dose prescribed;
- patient frequency and pattern of actual dosing;
- patient absorption, distribution, metabolism, and excretion of the drug, its metabolites, and contaminants;
- patient diet composition and pattern of eating, position, sleep, and activity;
- patient circadian, menstrual, and other biorhythms;
- patient gender, age, race, height, obesity, and muscle mass; and
- patient drug metabolising enzyme status as influenced by genes, illness, diet, concomitant drugs, and perfusion.

New customers demand re-evaluation of our quality metrics

In the past the customer was perceived to be regulatory authorities, who demanded a *"p <.05"* result, but accepted a small homogeneous population. Today the *customer* is recognised as being the *patient* as well as the patient's family, the patient's employer, and the payer for health care. These customers care, not what results have been achieved under optimal conditions in ideal compliant patients, but what will happen to them. To provide this information, to optimise therapy in the *"real"* population of customers, and to avoid predictable serious adverse events, we must today include in each protocol as many diverse patients as can be studied safely.

Protocols, especially in Phase III and IV, should be naturalistic, resembling to the fullest possible extent the actual use of the product expected in the world marketplace. Publications of *efficacy* and *safety* should emphasise the extent to which they are expected to predict *efficiency* in actual use.

Quality today is defined by the *patient*. Is the patient more interested in the millimoles of cholesterol or the future risk of myocardial infarction? Does the customer prefer the immediate risks of hypoglycaemia with "tight" insulin therapy to the greater likelihood of remote diabetic " ...opathies?" How does the patient compare the millimetres reduction in blood pressure measured during a visit to the white-robed high priest of sphygmomanometry to the cost and dys-ease of blood pressure medications *versus* the potential future reduction of the risk of stroke and renal failure?

Dose–utility instead of dose–response

What is the overall quality of life of the patient? What utilities does the patient assign to the cost and inconvenience of therapy, the potential and perceived benefits, and the potential and perceived adverse events?

Utilities can be assessed by patients in various ways if they are fully informed. They may be given rating scales, assign preferences in an analytical hierarchy, choose the years of life they would give up in a poorer state of health to achieve improved health for a shorter period. As compared with a certainty of a defined health state, such as the current one, the patient may estimate the probability of the worst possible health state he/she would accept for the complementary probability of the best possible health state. Such methods redefine *responses* as patient *utilities* and allow definition of population variables that influence the *dose–utility relationship*.

Lilly strategy

Lilly has revised its clinical trial strategies to assess multicultural dose–response effects, including quality of life, in large scale global clinical trials. Some principles are:

- conducting almost entirely dose–response trials, from the first patients, in which each patient is allocated randomly to one of several possible doses which include comparator drug(s) or placebo or both;
- conducting prospective trials in which the patient, investigator, and Lilly are blinded to the allocations of therapy until an official data lock and unblinding of the Lilly analyst;
- ensuring minimal exclusion of patients, early incorporation of women, and inclusion of all ages that are safe for study (often with no age limit);
- conducting trials with the same protocol in 20+ countries simultaneously including North America, Europe, Israel, South Africa, and Australia;
- utilising common global definitions of efficacy variables, adverse event classification terms (COSTART), patient instructions, investigator instructions, and data collection instruments;
- capturing every datum on each patient in standardised formats with exquisite validation in a single global database (rendering paper records meaningless);

- conducting one complex analysis of very large trials with careful study of the influence of identifiable factors;
- using *pre hoc* stratification wherever possible; and
- reinterpreting the clinical laboratory test results analysed by the patient's age, gender, racial origin, smoking, and ethanol use in comparison with reference data on results and their changes from baseline in 20 000 patients taking placebo.

Currently, a global trial of a new rapid-acting human insulin analogue is being conducted in 21 countries utilising the Clinical Trial Management data system that performs high-level edits on data entry soon after the patient visit. This rapid capture of validated data enhances safety in non-uniform or fragile patients.

Loracarbef

An example of these strategies is the clinical trials of the recently-approved oral carbacephem antimicrobial, loracarbef. Premarketing trials were conducted in 20 countries by 578 investigators treating 13 000 patients ranging in age from 0.3 to 94 years who generated one million routine laboratory test results. Safety data were analysed across all patients treated in Occidental countries who were on similar or identical protocols.

In these clinical trials there were profound differences in the reporting of adverse events between major Occidental countries. The frequency of patients reporting adverse events, most of which were probably not related to the antimicrobial, was greatest in Canada and decreased progressively in Sweden, US, Finland, France, UK, Germany, Italy (Zerbe *et al.*, 1992). Such four-fold differences in adverse event reporting rates make analysis of pooled data difficult. The rates of adverse events reported in labelling should specify the method of data collection and the cultures and ethnic origins of patients included in the tabulation.

Ethnic differences in duodenal ulcer treatment

Ethnic differences were also observed in testing the acute healing of duodenal ulcers demonstrated by gastroscopy. Acute healing of duodenal ulcers was least frequent during placebo treatment of Caucasian patients and on nizatidine therapies it was least frequent in patients of African origin. At lower doses healing rates were somewhat greater in patients of Hispanic origin. Duodenal ulcer recurrence was least in Caucasians treated with either placebo or nizatidine, but recurrence was greater in placebo-treated patients of African origin (Cloud and Enas, 1985–1986).

Fluoxetine trials in four diseases

Of particular interest are multicultural global studies of fluoxetine which were prospective, triple-blind, randomised, and highly validated. The results noted below are from 2539 patients treated for depression, bulimia, obsessive–compulsive disorder (OCD), or obesity with daily fluoxetine doses of 0 and usually 60 mg/d and at least two intermediate doses per disease of 5, 10, 20 or 40 mg/d. All trials began with a period of observation during patient-blinded treatment with placebo.

Efficacy was dose-dependent for each illness, but maximum effects were observed at different doses. The optimal single daily dose for depression was about 20 mg. OCD efficacy was substantial at 20 mg but increased further at 60 mg. There were few differences in OCD efficacy, as measured by the Yale Brown Obsessive Compulsive Score (YBOCS) decrement at endpoint, among ages (dichotomised at 50 y/o) and gender. Weight loss in obesity was greatest in patients of African origin and was both dose-dependent and obesity-dependent with weight loss being greatest at 60 mg daily in patients with body mass indices greater than $40 \, kg/m^2$. Bulimia showed the greatest dose-dependence with slight effect at 20 mg but substantial effects at 60 mg.

In each of these trials there was benefit of studying the entire *population distribution* of each variable. In all trials some patients had increased severity of the disease while treated with placebo or fluoxetine. In all trials some patients responded well to placebo. The effects when expressed as means or medians did reflect the overall effects, but a physician using the drug would obtain valuable information from the total patient population distribution of effects.

The percentage of patients stopping the trial for adverse events decreased with increasing dose in obesity. Discontinuations increased slightly with dose in bulimia but more profoundly in depression and OCD.

Treatment-emergent signs and symptoms

Treatment-emergent signs and symptoms (TESS) are those that appear after an initial placebo period or those whose severity increase after the visit at which allocation to different therapies is made. Patients with depression reporting at least one TESS increased with increasing dosage, but ethnic origin was unrelated. Patients with obesity treated with placebo had TESS frequencies similar to patients with depression, but there was little increased frequency of TESS reporting with higher doses. Slightly more patients with bulimia reported TESS, but the greatest dose-dependency of TESS reporting was in patients with OCD. Patients of African origin with OCD had the highest rates of TESS reporting, but race had little effect compared with diagnosis and dose in other illnesses.

Treatment and discontinuation, emerging and improving, signs and symptoms

In addition to TESS it is important to examine treatment improving signs and symptoms (TISS), discontinuation emergent signs and symptoms (DESS), and discontinuation improving signs and symptoms (DISS). For example, in obesity treated for longer periods, the TESS that are more frequent with fluoxetine than placebo include nausea, somnolence, tremor, and asthenia. TESS more frequent on placebo include rhinitis, depression, abdominal pain, and constipation. TISS more frequent with fluoxetine than placebo include oedema, polyuria, and thirst.

DESS more frequent with fluoxetine include increased appetite, depression, and sinusitis. DISS reported more often with fluoxetine include sleep disorder, somnolence, tremor, asthenia, and insomnia (Goldstein and Wilson, 1993). Such careful classification of adverse events occurring in these four modes helps confirm casual relationships with the drug and dose and indicate the value of post-treatment blinded periods of observation during placebo.

Insomnia TESS reporting was more common in bulimia than depression, with slight dose-dependence. Patients of African origin had greater reporting rates in OCD and obesity with those rates being especially large in OCD and more modest in obesity. Sweating TESS reporting was especially common in patients of African origin with OCD or depression at high doses. Otherwise there was little dose or racial dependence. Libido diminution was prominent in OCD and at higher doses especially in patients of African origin. This was also true at 60 mg doses in obese patients of African origin, but other groups had similar reporting rates with only modest dose-dependence. Yawning reporting rates increased substantially with dosing in OCD and bulimia, but there was little dose-dependence in obesity or depression and little distinction based on racial origin. Dry mouth showed the greatest racial effect with higher frequency of reporting in all four diseases in patients of African origin. In Caucasians there was little dose-dependence in depression, obesity, or bulimia, but a more prominent dose effect in OCD.

Large, single, multicultural rather than small, multiple clinical trials

These observations of triple-blinded dose–response studies of a single drug in four distinct diseases illustrate the interactions of key factors such as dose, disease, ethnic origin, as well as age and gender.

Meta-analyses focus on the average effect rather than on the whole population, and therefore neglect some of the most significant utilities and dys-utilities. Is there an example of a meta-analysis that examines dose–response relationships, the effects of age, or describes the 2% most deviant patients?

The average NDA now submitted to the FDA contains about 80 clinical protocols (Mocniak, 1992). A far more meaningful study design is to use only a few protocols, one if possible, for all patients with appropriate *pre-hoc* stratification. This permits sophisticated analysis of the influence of patient characteristics on the safety and efficacy results.

Conclusion

Substantial differences in efficacy and adverse events can be noted among Occidental patients of Caucasian, African, or Hispanic origin. Such relationships are complex and may depend on the diagnosis and dose as well as on gender and age. These observations suggest that estimations of efficiency in general use are best made from large global trials that admit widely diverse patients and analyse results carefully by many defined factors. It may be suggested that the "average" patient contributes little to the understanding of dose–utilities, as utilities are especially strong at the extremes of the populations. Therefore one should strive for enrolment of diverse populations and suppress the enrolment and observations of "average" patients.

Acknowledgements

The contribution of Ashbrook E, Beasley CM Jr, Cloud ML, Conforti PM, Enas GG, Enas NH, Goldstein DJ, Holman SL, Kotsanos JG, Levine LR, Masica DN, Rampey AH Jr, Roback PJ, Sanger TM, Sayler ME, Talbott MW, Taylor RE, Thompson VL., Tollefson GD, Wernicke JF, Wheedon DE, Wilson MG, Zerbe RL to this paper is gratefully acknowledged.

References

Cloud ML, Enas NH (1985–1986). Personal communication.

Goldstein DJ, Wilson MG (1993). Adverse event frequencies generate hypotheses of efficacy and safety. *Clin Pharmacol Ther* **54**: 245–51.

Mocniak N (1992). Acting Deputy Associate Commissioner for Planning and Evaluation, FDA, personal communication 22 Dec 92.

Zerbe RL, Conforti PM, Enas GG, Johns D Jr, and Martindale SJ (1992). Assessing country differences in clinical trial adverse event reporting. Presented at the Drug Information Association Meeting, San Diego, USA, 10 June 1992.

19
General discussion and concluding remarks

MODERATOR: JEAN-MARC HUSSON

Introduction

I have been asked to chair the discussion for at least two reasons. Firstly, five years ago before going to Japan with the EC Pharmaceutical Mission, I, together with some colleagues from the French Industry, did a preliminary and pioneer retrospective study on 12 drugs of different classes developed both in Japanese and Caucasian subjects. We did not find real inter-ethnic differences in either pharmacokinetic or pharmacodynamic parameters, and some of the results were described in Dr Labbé's paper. Secondly, being the EFPIA Efficacy Task Force Leader for ICH2, I have a good general overview of the different topics under discussion for harmonisation through this process. In fact, the question of "Ethnic Factors in the Acceptability of Foreign Clinical Data" impinges on all the subjects discussed within the other Efficacy topics, but there will be a long way to go before achieving tangible results on the matter.

During this CMR Workshop, the main points on ethnic factors to be considered in the near future by both the authorities and the industry have been tackled. The real question is the relative importance for the development of new medicines of both extrinsic and intrinsic ethnic factors. Professor Jones and I have selected the highlights of the Workshop as the focus of this Session, which will lead to the identification of topics for future discussion.

Genetic polymorphism

Do we have the tools to detect genetic polymorphisms in pre-clinical or clinical studies?

Rawlins: A number of issues have been raised during this workshop. The first relates to ethnic differences, that may be due to important genetic factors that control drug metabolism and pharmacological response. However, the evidence presented here suggests that pharmacokinetic differences are not prominent – in fact they are difficult to find.

Wood: I do not know whether we have looked at the right things, or whether the sensitivity of the method is sufficient to detect a difference in pharmacokinetics. It would be reassuring if differences could be identified for a compound with a known difference in the isozymes between Japanese and Caucasians. If such differences cannot be detected, we are wasting a lot of money doing something that is still not going to pick up the difference. There is not much point in requiring testing in Japan because of pharmacogenetic differences, if in reality these studies do not pick up known pharmacokinetic differences. For example, did any of the studies done in an industrial setting pick up the known differences between Japanese and Caucasians for omeprazole, which has been studied in all three regions and is metabolised by the polymorphically distributed enzyme 2CMP? Most of the data relates to pharmacokinetics and it ought to be possible to detect the major difference in the incidence of poor metaboliser phenotypes between the two populations if the method works. If it cannot be detected, that means that there is a large chance that a significant difference will be missed. Even if the pharmacokinetic difference is demonstrated in this kind of study, it may have no clinical significance for omeprazole. However, it may have considerable clinical significance for diazepam, for example, which is also metabolised by that system.

Wong: Omeprazole has been marketed in Japan for three years. From what I know, the clinical assessment done in Japan is somewhat different if you look at ulcer healing, because the parameters used for ulcer healing are different from those used in other countries. Therefore it is rather difficult to just look at the efficacy from the Japanese data. Drawing on experience with other populations, we have accumulated more than 3000 patients' data in my databank in Singapore, mainly from south Asians and Chinese

Asians. The efficacy at 20 mg of omeprazole shows similar healing rates compared to the European data. So in terms of efficacy, one would say that at the same dose level it is equal. Similarly, we have not seen any differences in terms of adverse events. In fact we do see a lower incidence of side-effects recorded in our patients which is again perhaps due to medical practices.

Davies: That does not mean that the methods are inadequate, it means for the vast majority of drugs, the dose–response is such that differences due to pharmacokinetics are not picked up. A drug which has a steep dose–response curve, and a genetic polymorphism in its elimination is unlikely to be widely used.

Balant: The question is what are we looking at and how should we look for it? I would distinguish between known polymorphisms and all those that are unknown. Professor George mentioned that when he was studying bufuralol, a new medication in hypertension, two volunteers had side-effects and vomiting, which we now know to be the classical effect of bufuralol in a poor metaboliser. He had included these two patients because they were intolerant to debriso-quine, and he did not know at the time that there was a common problem. So there is the whole problem of the unknown, and we should not extrapolate the methodologies derived from the known polymorphisms to the unknown situations we may encounter in the future.

Wood: Professor George has shown that there may be an inter-ethnic difference in the metabolism of nifedipine between what he called south Asians and Caucasians. If that is extrapolatable to all 3A4 substrates, then that is a huge issue. Dr Balant is right, there are other isozymes which we know very little about.

Jones: Dr Breimer presented data on ethnic difference in the metabolism of debrisoqine and mephenytoin. The problem I have is knowing whether it is genetic or whether it is due to environmental factors.

Breimer: The debrisoquine/sparteine polymorphism is very insensitive to environmental factors. In other words, it can hardly be induced – it can be inhibited, but in most of the reported studies this was taken into consideration. I am quite sure that in these particular cases you are dealing with a genetic situation which is now substantiated with genotyping.

Wood: Chinese and Japanese subjects living in the US certainly show the same distribution for mephenytoin and debrisoquine polymorphism. When we tried to look for environmental differences, the only obvious one we could find in the diet was that Chinese consistently eat more rice even in the US than Caucasians. I think debrisoquine is more easily inducible *per se*, however the data that shows it is not inducible is somewhat poorer. I believe it is based on the fact that extensive metabolisers cannot be turned into poor metabolisers on the basis of their metabolic ratio, but you clearly can induce metabolic clearance and we have good data to show this. I think we have become acclimatised to seeing an excellent correlation between different probes. When we look at drugs and their polymorphisms, we always find it shows debrisoquine metabolic ratio against drug X. But if we move into looking at a non-polymorphic enzyme, we cannot find a correlation between different probes. That may reflect the fact that instead of looking at a spread that goes over a number of orders of magnitude such as you see with a polymorphism, with a non-polymorphic enzyme you do not have nearly such a wide range. So before we make a leap of faith and say X is an excellent probe for cytochrome $P_{450, 3A4}$ or whatever, we should be sure the probe correlates with other drugs and enzymes.

What is the importance of this problem for drug development?

Balant: I will comment from a European stance, which may be only a partial view. With the exception of perhaps renal function, the variability of every elimination mechanism is under genetic control. Pharmacogenetic variability is a source of variability like any other and has to be treated in exactly the same way. The advantage with known polymorphisms is that there are ways to be pro-active in order to detect potential problems during drug development. Our experience in Europe is mainly in one ethnic group as far as drug development is concerned, and we are not usually exploring the consequences of potential inter-ethnic differences. We have devised a strategy for exploring the relevance of known polymorhisms in drug metabolism from *in vitro* systems to full scale clinical trials. This topic has been discussed extensively and published in the *European Journal of Clinical Pharmacology*. The attitude we have had is to try not to make a blockade to drug development because of interesting scientific problems, and 12 countries in Europe have agreed that this is a reasonable stance, as discussed in a Consensus

Conference held under the auspices of the European Co-ordinated Action (COST B1).

Wood: I agree. Actually knowing the isozyme responsible for the metabolism of the drug is a huge advantage, as it is possible to predict which drugs are likely to interact with it, both in terms of inhibition and induction. That is going to make an enormous difference to cost as it will not be necessary to study an encyclopaedia of drugs chosen randomly, or because for historical reasons the FDA liked certain drugs to be looked at. It is possible to actually select drugs in a more rational fashion. On the other hand, we ought not to be too self-confident about what we know about polymorphism. Everyone has talked about isozymes in terms of 2D6 and 2CMP, but these are not even the most important for drug metabolism. 3A is much more important, and there is some data to suggest that there may be ethnic differences in 3A. So I think we ought not to get ourselves locked into too self-confident a position based on our 1993 knowledge, when that may change over the next few years. It is inconceivable to me that knowledge of the enzyme responsible for drug metabolism is not a major plus in rational drug development – it is certainly not a negative.

Husson: Professor Naito, what is the attitude in Japan?

Naito: We have not yet decided any new policy based on our recent new data on pharmacokinetics. Because of the amount of data requested, in our study we have no acetylator drug data, and just one or two of the drugs could be subject to genetic polymorphism. So we feel it is too early to have any conclusion from our preliminary analyses, as more data is needed on drugs metabolised by a route governed by genetic polymorphism.

Rawlins: I agree with what Dr Wood has said, particularly because of the value in relation to interactions. The other area we have rather forgotten is that there are also pharmacodynamic genetic polymorphisms and although we know little about it or its implications at the present time, I suspect that by the year 2000 we may well know a great deal more and that also may be a useful tool in terms of drug development.

Husson: There are differences between populations concerning the plasma concentration of some transport system proteins, for example α_1-glycoprotein. What is the importance of ethnic differences in such proteins and what are the consequences for the bioavailability of drugs?

Edwards: Low levels of such proteins result in free drug circulating, which may have implications for toxic effects. The reality is, however, we do not see much clinical difference and although the academic reports are interesting, the clinical data is the important part. There are some drugs clearly where there are implications for α_1 protein, for example, drugs such as the phenothiazines, tricyclics and dysopyramide agents, as opposed to effects of metabolism or pharmacodynamics such as the hypertensive agents which are less effective in black populations, and black populations tend to be more resistant to calcium channel blockers and β-blockers. Apart from that, there is a very limited spectrum of real differences in clinical activity.

Breimer: I tend to agree with Dr Edwards. However, I would be interested to see more studies being performed on activities of the principal systems because I do not think that we have addressed the question of transport systems to a sufficient extent to judge whether or not it is clinically relevant. I also have to admit that we may not, until now, have had the right tools to study that in a relevant *in vivo* situation. But I would not be surprised if that type of protein carrier would exhibit a large degree of inter-subject variability with potential clinical implications.

Levy: Coming back again to whether ethnic differences are real in terms of clinical outcome, Dr Edwards suggested this may not be the case in most situations. But I can think of two situations where these differences may occur. Firstly, if a patient is switched between generics, there may be a small difference in bioavailability which, if super-imposed on ethnic and racial difference, may collude to produce a real clinical difference. Another is in some situations where different drugs of a class are substituted for each other in a stabilised patient, so-called therapeutic substitution which is now an active policy in some countries. One of the drugs may operate on one metabolic pathway and the other may not, so there may be genetic polymorphisms involved. It may therefore be necessary to make a rapid dose adjustment to keep the proper clinical dose.

Balant: We systematically monitor tricyclic antidepressant drug concentrations in patients in Geneva and we have some cases where patients are poor metabolisers of debrisoquine and need for example only 25 mg of clomipramine per day instead of 100–125 mg usually prescribed. If one gives these patients the normal dose, they would be on toxic levels. Some patients tend not to respond to the medication when the concentrations get too high, and when one decreases the concentration, they improve. This emphasises that if one is testing new substances it is crucial to have concentration measurements. If one just increases dosing to find maximum efficacy and safe dose, without knowledge of blood concentrations one might reach very wrong conclusions.

Breimer: Does that not also lead to the conclusion that although polymorphisms are very interesting from a scientific point of view, it may not be any more relevant than any other factor? In other words, we jump on it because we can measure or assess it, but it is the variability *per se* and quality of variability which is interesting to us, and to what extent it relates to different ethnic populations. But whether or not there are 2–3% or even 10% more poor metabolisers, in a certain population, is not a major issue.

Dollery: I wanted to make a very similar point because if you are actually setting the price for your drug you might be very interested in the average dose that will be used kinetically. But if you are in a position of treating patients you should be more interested in the range of individual dose requirements. It seems to me that with practically everything, with one or two exceptions, the range of individual dose requirements within a country or within an ethnic group is wider than the difference is between countries and ethnic groups. Therefore, I would have thought that a physician should not use the average recommended dose in all patients.

Representativeness of the test population in comparison to the potential marketed population

How can a more diverse population be obtained without extending the overall development time?

Thompson: No one should be excluded from clinical trials unless there is a very reasonable belief that there is a safety concern, which in my experience does not happen very often. I do not understand why there should, for example, be an upper age limit for clinical trials, or why women who are not likely to become pregnant need to be excluded from trials if they consent. The ideal is to have the most diversity possible, and I therefore find it difficult to understand why there appears to be an attempt within ICH to obtain agreement that there is no need to do clinical trials in all three major cultural areas – why should people from Japan, North America and Europe not be specifically included in clinical trials? Certainly if their utility functions are assessed they will be different, independently of whether there are any differences in drug concentrations.

Rawlins: For the sake of discussion, I would like to suggest another way of looking at this issue. It could be argued with equal cause that the initial studies should be conducted in a relatively homogeneous population in whom there is less likelihood of causing damage than in a wider group. This would proceed via a process of gradualism, and at the time of first licensing, doctors should be informed of the type of population that has been treated. I am not suggesting that the indication should be restricted, but doctors should be aware that the first clinical trials have been drawn from a specific homogeneous population, and they need to take considerable care if they go outside this group.

Jones: I think that is an excellent idea, provided it is not used carte blanche to get off label use. It sorts out the second part of the issue, and allows both therapeutic and commercial benefits to be reaped in a reasonable space of time. If it is done properly, with follow up Phase IIIb and IV studies, that is probably a very good method.

Husson: Professor Naito, do you want to react on these questions?

Naito: I would like to have a definition of "representative".

Husson: This is a very good point, which was raised in Dr Thompson's paper. Do we have in the database during drug development the type of patients that will be exposed to the drug after marketing? In other words, we are really selecting patients for drug development purposes. They are not taking any other drugs and we minimise the number of drug interactions. What is the real situation when the drug is on the market?

Naito: I understand the concept, but in reality it is very difficult because the drug will be used after marketing in people with different kinetics and genetics, and it is not possible to find a representative population to test the drug. I think when we do clinical tests for drug development, maybe we cannot help limiting the subjects.

Husson: You would like to limit the use of the drug after approval, as suggested by Professsor Rawlins, but then you do not have the right to use the drug in other types of populations, at least at the beginning of product life.

Naito: Sometimes that would be necessary, but I do not think it is necessary to include always all races when we carry out clinical studies for drug development.

Are studies in specific ethnic populations necessary?

Jones: Let me be more pragmatic. Taking Professor Rawlins' suggestion that conducting the first studies in a well defined homogeneous population, and bringing in others at a later stage, is not a bad way forward, what is a homogeneous population for commercial reasons? I would suggest that it would be inappropriate and not practicable to carry out the studies in every single group, but you would want the bulk of the populations to be represented in the first sample. In North America that would be largely Caucasian, black and Hispanic, but how would you identify Hispanic? How many more sub-groups should be included? It will depend largely on the drug.

Wood: It seems to me we are getting way beyond the data. What we are asked to do is to not exclude people from studies, and the idea that it is necessary to have a quota in studies seems to me ridiculous. There needs to be some data-driven reason as to why we select a group. We need to have some index of suspicion that something is wrong in that group before we start to recruit quotas. Otherwise it seems to me a waste of time trying to prove that a particular racial group responds in a particular way. Of course that clue will only be obtained if a reasonably heterogeneous population is included, and I think clearly there are two things driving that. One is science, which is probably very small. The other is politics, and that is not necessarily satisfied by checking some box that the study includes people of any particular racial group.

Jones: If data generated in Europe and North America can be used in those two geographies, then it seems to me that Caucasian and black populations have been covered by first attempt, and Japan will be separate for the foreseeable future. It is then a question of what scientific parameters drive you – we want to do more than that initially. Beyond that it is really a commercial decision as to which other groups are included in the trials deliberately to create a database. The question really is, do you exclude these additional groups, or do you just allow them to become part of the database as experience with the drug increases? I would let them become part of the database, but I think I would deliberately go out and try to get sufficient black and Caucasian subjects.

Recording of race

Rawlins: At the Committee on Safety of Medicines we have discussed whether ethnicity should be included in the Yellow Card ADR reporting scheme, and we have been ambivalent over it. It could be useful, particularly in a multicultural society such as the UK, but on the other hand, there are problems. Firstly, there is a lot of intermarriage and it would be difficult to describe some of the categories, and, secondly, it might cause offence.

Gennery: In clinical investigations in the US the recording of race has been routinely required for years now – have they found that to be of value, or is it, as many of us suspect, pretty useless?

Wood: It is certainly used as a means for demonstrating inadequate representation of certain ethnic groups in the clinical studies. I am not sure it has shown much difference, although in some of the antihypertensive studies it has been useful, with the global names like black or Caucasian or Asian.

Balant: I think the question of how useful this information is will depend on the degree of integration of the population within the country. The more ethnic groups are integrated, the more difficult it will be to record the exact genetic background of each individual participating in clinical studies, and the less relevant the ethnicity will be as far as cultural factors are concerned.

Thompson: We have shown that this information is important in the interpretation of clinical laboratory data. We took 20 000 people who were on placebo, enrolled in a trial where one would not have anticipated a major abnormality in the routine 36 clinical laboratory tests. There were five major demographic characteristics which highly significantly altered the population distribution of values of these analytes: race, gender, age, smoking and drinking. We tested self-reported race in several ways, and the most powerful dichotomi-sation was between Caucasian and non-Caucasian. We have now divided laboratory values into 32 separate distributions, depending on the dichotomised value of the five variables. There is a ten-fold difference in the upper 99 percentile point for creatine kinase value between the highest (a young, black, smoking, drinking male), and an older woman who does not admit to smoking or drinking. So I think that in just interpreting routine laboratory values it is worth collecting some of these data.

Voith: I would like to return to the earlier discussion and ask how the industry or regulators foresee labelling of the drugs even if all this knowledge is accumulated? I am very supportive of the sugges-tion of studying the drug in ethnic populations as much as possible, but how do you foresee labelling of these drugs? In Japan the population is very homogeneous, as opposed to Canada and the United States which are multi-racial. Should we tell our physicians, for example in British Columbia where there is a large Chinese population, about differences observed in clinical trials between Caucasian and Chinese patients?

Thompson: There are two steps, the first is to actually study the diverse population. The second step is to include in labelling those things which are significant. If they are not significant there is no problem, and if they are significant there is also no problem because they will have to be included in the label anyway. So it is not necessary to needlessly increase the size of the label. The way I suggest amending the label now is to include the explicit statement describing the population from which the data were obtained.

Should women be included in Phase I studies?
Should Phase III studies be performed in pregnant women?

Thompson: Dr Edwards, what do you think the primary bar is in putting fecund women into early trials? It has been suggested to me that it is not in fact a regulatory prohibition but it is, in the US, the liability you will run into, in the sense that the unborn fetus cannot have its rights taken away by anyone.

Edwards: I also serve on the Institute of Medicines Committee, commissioned by the National Institute of Health, which deals with legal and ethical questions involved with exposure of women during clinical trails. We have several lawyers on this panel and they have been making the very strong point that while the fetus is a potential person, it does not have the legal rights of an actual person. They argue that to avoid medication because of the possibility that a woman might become pregnant and that pregnancy might result in a live infant, puts the women's rights beyond that of a possible human being. However, in clinical studies they are pushing to make a recommendation to recruit pregnant women into all therapeutic studies because they do not wish to exclude them. This should not apply to Phase I, when you are looking at dosages with no potential benefit, unless it is in a disease area such as AIDS or cancer.

Marshall: If we start to include women in Phase I studies, what effect do you think that is going to have on the timing of the toxicology studies and reproductive toxicology studies?

Thompson: Lilly has been putting women who cannot become pregnant in Phase I trials, but it does require doing more teratology studies. I do not see any problem there, but the idea of putting in a woman who is pregnant and putting the fetus at risk I think is unusual.

Jones: If we are talking about drug development, from research into clinical pharmacology *per se* it is a pragmatic issue, based on how much drug is to be made, when to start reproductive studies to get agreement before continuing or terminating development. We use men as the prime target for the first phase. If women are recruited into trials that will add a lot of cost to drug development. We really should be resisting that in terms of benefit to society in the shorter term, otherwise it will delay our programmes.

Wood: What people are saying is that women should not be excluded – that is subtly different from the interpretation that is being put on it here. In the past we have deliberately excluded women, now the NIH and the agency are saying that should stop. You will not be funded to do a study if you say you are deliberately going to exclude women from the study, unless you have got some reason. If you are testing a drug as a treatment for prostatic cancer, then it is perfectly reasonable to say you are only going to look at men. What was said was that women have been poorly represented in therapeutic trials, and in Phase III efficacy studies. That should not be extrapolated to equal participation in Phase I studies. It seems inconceivable to me that any Institutional Review Board in the USA would approve a study that was going to give a Phase I drug to a pregnant woman.

Voith: I spoke to a number of my colleagues, and their viewpoint is that women are very often under-represented in clinical trials, and many of these are investigating conditions for which women should be participating in clinical trials. We also get similar feedback from our clinicians, who have difficulty collecting sufficient data in women because we only allow post-menopausal or sterile women to participate in clinical trials. I do not think that any regulatory agency would demand that equal numbers of men and women should be included in clinical trials, but the exclusion criteria should not be as strict as they have been in the past. The issue of women also applies to safety. For example, for a drug which might cause amenorrhea, this effect will be much less likely to be detected in a six or eight week clinical trial than in a six months clinical trial. However, there are very limited data in women available from long-term clinical trials in the field of psychiatry. So if you only have male and post-menopausal females included, and I am thinking of a particular experience that I recently had, then you might miss some of these adverse reactions.

Rawlins: I do not think that studies deliberately in pregnant women are appropriate, otherwise they become human teratology studies and I would wish to have nothing to do with it. What one should do is to make much better use of the information that is lost. In other words there will be circumstances where either accidentally or deliberately pregnant women are exposed to drugs in the routine course of clinical practice and we ought to develop better methods of capturing those sort of episodes. The other thing is children. We are in danger of creating a new generation of therapeutic orphans because very few new drugs, for understandable reasons, are tested in children and yet my paediatric colleagues use most new drugs in children, ground up by the pharmacists and given as a guessed dose. We really do need to either capitalise on those sorts of individual experiments that are going on all over Europe and North America to find out what is happening, or in some way get our act together to ensure that we can make the best possible arrangements for children. I do not think I have an easy solution, but I think it is a very, very important issue.

Tolerance and safety issues

Dose titration versus fixed dose

Husson: Dose titration versus fixed dose is a part of medical practice, but it is a really big issue for all of us, not only at industry level, but concerning the clinicians and the authorities.

Walker: Are any industry people incorporating the type of approach described in Dr Balant's paper into their Phase III studies at the present time?

Gennery: I think in the US Benoxaprofen Phase III studies we actually did plasma levels on every visit, and that was a drug with a very long half-life. There was really no correlation between those levels and side-effects. I do not recall that we ever tried to analyse it for efficacy. That single experience made me suspicious of this process, as not producing anything terribly worthwhile.

Jones: My immediate reaction is how many drugs can you be assured have a good correlation between plasma level concentrations and clinical effect? For example, 5-lipoxygenase inhibitors can be washed out of the body in a few hours, but lipoxygenase inhibition can still be detected for 24 or 48 hours. So what is the value of a plasma level profile? I do not even know what a 5 lipoxygenase inhibitor might do clinically, but if it does have an effect, it certainly is not necessarily going to be related to plasma levels. What about the site of activity of a drug? If we are testing an antiviral against HIV, lymph concentrations will probably be more important than plasma concentrations, and maybe even brain concentrations and not second compartments. If you look at the cascade of events that release, for example, nitric oxide in the body, what is the value of the plasma level of the drug against the eventual effect in something like stroke? So how many drugs are there with a really good correlation between clinical effect and plasma level parameters?

Balant: This is a question we are asked every time we speak about drug level monitoring. In Geneva, where the catchment area is 400 000, we are measuring about 3000 samples a year of anti-depressants and neuroleptics. The first answer is that there is no correlation to be found (in the statistical sense) between steady-state concentrations and, for example, a percentile decrease on a

Hamilton rating scale after four weeks of treatment. But what we know for sure, is that when the concentrations are really low, patients tend not to respond. If they are really high, patients tend to have side-effects which can be life endangering. That is all we are looking for – what we want to detect is subgroups who are really at risk. We are thus not looking for strict correlations or relations, we are looking for the detection of populations at risk. The approach I am trying to promote is really to detect those patients which will be the ones that will make the study fail, because of no efficacy, or those who will have serious side-effects and will increase the number of drop-outs.

Jones: We are not surprised by the use of plasma level monitoring for certain drugs, e.g. theophylline, phenytoin – there are many examples where you would not treat without routinely doing that, but only on the basis of drugs where you know there are some inter-relationships.

Rawlins: I have spent a good part of my life doing pharmacokinetics, and my department does about 10 000 routine samples a year, but I have to say the world is moving away from complicated healthcare technology towards simpler healthcare technology. Primary healthcare cannot cope with large quantities of plasma level monitoring, and we need to use drugs which do not require it. Maybe a small minority of people having transplants need a cyclosporin assay, and that sort of thing, but they are a minute proportion and I hate to think we are going along the route of having to license drugs for use at certain plasma concentrations, rather than certain dosages, because frankly I do not think healthcare deliverers are going to be able to do it.

Balant: I fully agree with you. First of all, I did not say that because one has been measuring blood concentrations during Phase III clinical trials, that blood level monitoring would be mandatory for therapeutic use. We are not going to prescribe concentrations for patients, even if information on dose–concentrations–response was obtained during drug development. The objection about healthcare is also absolutely correct. We look at concentration–response investigations as a research tool to compare and understand sources of variability, develop new methodologies for studying drugs. Accordingly, we are not advocating this type of approach as a general approach for the treatment of patients, but also as a research tool for the detection of sources of kinetic variability in relation to drug effects.

Jones: I take Professor Rawlins' point that he sees the world through an area of limited costs and more difficult reforms of assessing patients in terms of the diagnostic procedures, and I do not believe it practicable for the world to titrate patients as we do in our experiments in our scientific laboratories. The real nature of the world is not going to be that way, unless it is of course a specific disease area such as neuromuscular blockade or anaesthesia. So realistically, I regret to say, I think we will go for convenience wherever we can in each population.

Efficacy and adverse events

Jones: Professor Dollery, I think one of the reasons why physicians in Japan prescribe expensive new drugs, especially those which are "me-too" products, is probably associated with their reward system and not necessarily with additional benefit in terms of efficacy. Your analyses tended to look at efficacy as the prime factor, and I wonder if you also had a chance to look at safety as the prime factor?

Dollery: Both of those points are very well taken, and Dr Hirokawa and I have discussed them extensively but we do not have much data about them. What you say is true, I think not just of general practitioners but also of hospitals. Dr Hirokawa tells me that an important component of general practitioners' income in Japan is the difference between the wholesale and retail price of drugs and many patients who consult a doctor in Japan come away with a prescription for a number of drugs. They may get a drug which might irritate the stomach so they get a prescription for another which will prevent the first drug from irritating the stomach and so on, and often the prescriptions are for quite a short period of time so as to bring the patient back. He also says that he was surprised sitting in the Hammersmith Drug and Therapeutic Committee where we grill people who want to stock new drugs in the hospital. Although most general hospitals in Japan have a comparable committee, they are not so critical of new drugs because there is no exact budget for drugs and the price of drugs would be passed on in the billing system to the insurance carrier for the patient. In a sense the hospital also has an interest because they will also be charging the differences between the retail and wholesale price of the drug. So I am sure that those are powerful motivating forces, and Dr Hirokawa and many other Japanese friends have said to me that whereas in the West you might say the prime consideration is efficacy with an acceptable degree of safety, in Japan it is safety with an acceptable degree of efficacy so when there is a doubt they come down on the grounds of safety. I personally believe, and this is purely an opinion, that is the main reason the drug doses used in Japan are lower than in the West.

Breimer: If efficacy is not the primary issue in studies that were performed in Japan, but safety is, how actively is the assessment of safety actually pursued?

Dollery: The methods of assessing safety are really very similar to the methods used here, in other words, biochemical, haematological, urine monitoring, monitoring side-effects and so on. It sounds a very weak statement, but I think it is still true that the Japanese physicians and perhaps Japanese patients are very much imbued by the Hippocratic oath that "thou shalt do no harm" and that is the first priority. So when they are in the decision-making process on things like drug and dose that is at the foremost of their minds, whereas for a Western physician, efficacy might be at the forefront.

Rawlins: It is important that the studies reported during this workshop have demonstrated a rather significant reduction in adverse event reporting in Japanese populations, which is generally regarded as a common phenomenon. This is, in a sense, a cultural thing, as Japanese patients do not like to accuse their doctors of giving them side-effects.

Naito: That is partly true.

Jones: We should distinguish between serious adverse events, which do seem to be reported, and those which people would regard as almost background noise.

Edwards: Which are we going to take as the standard in terms of adverse reporting rates because, in looking at drugs across the world, there are vast variations in non-serious events between the different populations. The USA tends to be the highest together with Scandinavia, the UK and some parts of Europe tend to be about two-thirds, and Japan one-third to one-half, of that level seen in the US.

Rawlins: This is why different regulatory authorities form different trade-offs on risk and benefit, and on the same data they may come to different decisions.

Wong: With regard to reporting of adverse events, from my experience of running studies in Asia outside Japan, including mainly China, Taiwan, Korea and South Asia, there is a major problem in terms of communication. Hopefully this will be solved with the introduction of GCP in the South Asian countries. The English term "adverse events" is quite easily understandable, because there is a definition differentiating side-effects from adverse events. But the problem is that in a lot of Asian languages, and I think this includes Japanese, there is no difference between "adverse event" and "side-effect". For the physicians there is a responsibility to identify whether a symptom is regarded as a reasonable side-effect or not, and of course in the methodology of Western clinical trials anything that is considered as unusual is reported without assigning causality. This is not the case in the Asian culture or the language.

Voith: In the future we would like to see comparative tables of the incidence of side-effects in various ethnic populations. The current practice of pooling them may result in things being overlooked. As long as we realise what the incidence within the Asian population refers to, we can advise the physician. In listing adverse reactions it is important to first point out the clinically serious ones, even though sometimes the incidence is very low, or even without giving the actual incidence. This is the primary thing the physicians should be aware of, what can happen and what is most serious.

Utility assessment

Husson: So-called global utility assessment as proposed by our Japanese colleagues, is certainly a very important issue. We have to think of, besides clinical endpoints, primary or secondary endpoints and statistical significance of any results. We have to take into consideration all the atmosphere around the patients – the quality of life and other aspects – which are of real importance for the future.

Walker: Professor Naito, I was particularly interested in the overall assessment of utility in Japan, and its lack of value with regard to drug evaluation. When it comes to the submission of an NDA, what priority or value do the MHW actually put on this type of assessment?

Naito: In the primary evaluation, we approve the drug rather than the efficacy or safety data separately. We evaluate the utility data more heavily. But in the new general and statistics guidelines, and I chaired the groups that prepared them, I wanted to eliminate the utility evaluation system. Unfortunately I could not do that because beside me, there are several members of those groups (seven and ten, respectively), and only a few supported my suggestion. So I am afraid it will take a little more time to rationalise our evaluation system.

Papaluca: Do you have any experience in comparing your utility scale with some other Western or global assessment scales which are currently available?

Naito: Unfortunately I do not have the experience to compare those things.

Walker: Although I can see from Professor Naito the limitations of utility measures, I do think there is some value in being able to make an assessment of benefit versus risk in the way that was described. Rather than dismiss it I would like to look at some of the other methodologies that are available for making better benefit/risk assessments in this way and perhaps improve that.

Gennery: I agree. Before you throw this system out, I think it requires a little support, because with some refinement it may overcome some of the problems of ascribing adverse reactions in the wrong way. I suspect there is a kernel of value there that needs to be explored and developed and refined before it is discarded.

Acceptability of foreign data

Supportive and pivotal data

Walker: Dr Papaluca made the distinction between supportive and pivotal data. I would like to ask the other regulators whether foreign data from a study that conforms to appropriate study design, GCP and all the other criteria with which they judge studies, are accepted in their countries as pivotal or as supportive data. Secondly, have they ever approved products solely on the basis of foreign data, without any studies being conducted within their own country?

Voith: The distinction between pivotal and non-pivotal is very often made by the industry. However, to suggest that a study carried out in Canada and the United States would be regarded as pivotal, and studies conducted in Europe as non-pivotal, is ridiculous, and we look at both types of studies. I am sure that ten years ago a drug would have been licensed in Canada regardless of whether or not there were clinical trials in Canada, but I do not think that happens any more as we do not see new drug submissions in which there is no Canadian clinical trial. Recently there has been a change in the pharmaceutical industry and companies have made a major commitment to increase their clinical research in Canada. Furthermore we have excellent clinicians, and investigators. We like to see Canadians in clinical trials, but not to the extent of having "x number of patients from the Ottawa area" incorporated in these studies. In the future, clearly more clinical studies will become available which have been conducted in non-Caucasian populations, but to date we have seen very little of it. Probably the only exception was a new drug submission in our cardiovascular division which was reviewed very recently, in which approximately 1200 patients came from North America, approximately 800 patients from Europe and 500 patients from Japan.

Papaluca: If studies are carried out and reported in a manner consistent with the standards and the design of the trial itself, there is no problem. Major difficulties arise when the drug has been studied in way which is not standardised, which is not recognised. For example, there is no problem with a double blind, randomised pair of studies, or with an open, randomised well controlled study with blind evaluation of comparator. For a completely open study, not randomised, the acceptability of the clinical study is related to the protocol and to the way the trial is conducted and the reports are compared.

Wood: I think we are skirting around some of these issues by the use of euphemisms, like cultural differences, to cover up what is being projected as a parochial American point of view. In fact, there is a perspective that the documentation of many of the submissions that include foreign data is not as good as it would be with domestic data. However, there are two different issues, which I would like to distinguish. I think the data that is submitted for an NDA is almost always going to be OK, as it has been monitored by the company. Once the drug is on the market, however, the data to support a new indication sometimes comes from a major multinational trial which has been published, over which the company had no direct control. In that situation there is sometimes the perception that the studies are not the same and unfortunately the FDA is unable to validate the source document with monotonous regularity – going back and being unable to find the data. There are problems with pivotal studies that are not company-sponsored studies, which need to be addressed. There needs to be a recognition of the fact that even if they are published in the best journals, they are not acceptable if there is no back-up documentation.

Comparators

Rawlins: The question of comparators was raised, and the difficulties that regulators have in interpreting foreign data if there has been a comparator that is not used and not licensed in that particular country. Is the selection of appropriate comparators a serious problem for the industry?

Papaluca: In the past in Europe certainly we had differences, but now we are not in the same situation. Frankly speaking, apparently within the CPMP there are always two or three countries that remain quite reluctant to accept comparators which are not in their own market. However, the majority of countries accept comparators from different markets.

Gennery: If the comparator which is being used is not terribly well known in certain European states, part of the clinical expert report ought to be a discussion of the validity of the comparators.

Thompson: Lorabid had 13 000 patients on trial, about 8000 were required by the FDA for nine indications, but I think about 5000 were added by differences among European countries in duration of therapy and different comparator drugs. Some of the comparator drug differences are scientifically valid. For example, there is less β-lactamate resistance in Scandinavians. However, to get everything done across all the countries for nine indications resulted in 13 000 patients in trials, which is too many.

Issues for further discussion

Jones: In pulling together all that has been said during the Workshop, I believe there are a number of issues which require further discussion:

1. Should better routine probes be developed as markers of potential variability? There are 20 human forms of cytochrome P450 being characterised, each with distinct, but overlapping, substrate specificity. Perhaps it would help to have simple diagnostic tests that could be used in the clinical trial stage which, potentially, could be extended to routine practice. If so, what markers would be desirable and what additional research should be carried out?

2. Although there is a considerable body of data on genetic and ethnic differences often it is on very small numbers of subjects, typically, in some of the studies, for six or eight subjects. There are larger meta analyses, but should an attempt be made to network some very large pre-planned studies in this area and, if so, how would they be designed, what would be the top three chosen, and who would pay to do it?

3. There still seem to be many local diseases such as "heavy legs", "liverishness" and "acid stomach". Are any groups of therapeutic specialists attempting to see whether these can be given some kind of lexicon, some kind of commonality, so that in speaking internationally with colleagues, everyone knows what is meant by these various descriptors?

4. Since we use different doses as an important means of adjusting for variability, whether it is genetic or ethnic, are we moving to an international practice of dose tailoring or not; should we, could we, and so on? As an aside, although not the subject of this Workshop, Dr Breimer did advise us that whereas these considerations relate to drugs, we really have to remember there are also similar considerations applying to other materials and xenobiotics in general.

5. Dr Edwards stated that clinical studies for regulatory submissions are growing larger, taking longer, costing more, and Dr Patterson demonstrated some of the times and costs. Many of the studies are to accommodate ethnic or regional differences, and there will be further recommendations in the future. This raises questions: is this the right direction; at what stage should

this data be obtained (Phase III, IIIb or IV); can we influence the extent to which studies should be extended, or, in reality, is this an inexorable expansion of the length of a clinical programme? Dr Edwards pointed out that the ICH Expert Working Group will present recommendations at ICH3. These may include deliberate planning to involve females and the major racial groups in clinical studies, recording menses data, deliberately looking for differences in the data rather than just the outlying data, looking at trend analysis by gender and, if sufficient, by racial group and finally including in publications discussing differences, the number of patients per group and outlining the importance of relying on only statistically significant data. The main problem is what is meant by "major racial groups" on an international basis? Dr Edwards explained very clearly how that could be confusing within one country, North America. How will that translate when acquiring data on an international basis, including, for example, the EC, Asia, the Middle East, Africa, the Caribbean, Latin America, South-East Asia, China, and so on? Can these effects be sufficiently covered in a major multinational international study? How do you select on the basis of ethnic groups and how are these planned?

6.   Dr Breimer commented that governments do not realise or perhaps do not want to hear that people vary, they need choice, they need selection. By this we mean not just different doses, but different drugs. This clearly involves the political areas of formulary, pricing control and selection. Dr Breimer also stated: *"The existence of genetic polymorphism should be considered as a special case of inter-subject variability and should not be a reason per se for not developing or not marketing a drug, unless of course drug safety and/or efficacy could be highly compromised ... After all, many clinically important drugs are on the market which exhibit this type of polymorphism and it was only recognised by a retrospective study. I think we could over emphasise problems at the early stage when in reality we live with them and we have very efficient medicines as a result".*

Appendix
Workshop participants

Dr G Ahr, Clinical Pharmacology Department, Bayer AG, Germany

Dr R Ayesh, Head of Clinical Unit, BIBRA Toxicology International, UK.

Dr L P Balant, Head of the Clinical Research Unit, Psychiatric University Institutions of Geneva, Switzerland.

Dr A Barner, Director of Medicine Division, Boëhringer Ingelheim GmbH, Germany

Professor D D Breimer, Professor of Pharmacology and Director of Research, Leiden/Amsterdam Center for Drug Research, Leiden University, The Netherlands

Dr C Broome, Group Director of Clinical Pharmacology, General and AI Medicine, SmithKline Beecham Pharmaceuticals, UK

Professor D S Davies, Director of the Department of Clinical Pharmacology, Royal Postgraduate Medical School, University of London, UK

Professor Sir Colin Dollery, Dean, Royal Postgraduate Medical School, University of London, UK

Ms E Donnelly, Director and Senior Vice President, Transnational Regulatory Affairs & Compliance, SmithKline Beecham Pharmaceuticals

Dr L D Edwards, Assistant Vice President, International Clinical Research, Hoffmann-La Roche Inc, USA

Dr M J Ferris, Director of Japan Liaison Development, Glaxo Group Research Limited, UK

Dr B A Gennery, General Manager, Otsuka Pharmaceutical Company Limited, UK

Professor C F George, Professor of Clinical Pharmacology, University of Southampton, UK

Dr C Harvey, former Senior Research Associate, Centre for Medicines Research, UK

Dr J Henderson, Senior Vice President - Medical, Pfizer Pharmaceuticals Inc, USA

Dr K Hirokawa, Research Fellow, Department of Clinical Pharmacology, Royal Postgraduate Medical School, University of London, UK

Dr J-M Husson, Head of Medical Affairs, Pharma Policy Direction, Roussel Uclaf, France

Professor T M Jones, Director Research, Development and Medical, Wellcome Foundation Limited, UK

Dr E Labbé, Medical Director for Japan, Synthelabo Recherche, France

Dr R A Levy, Vice President, Scientific Affairs, National Pharmaceutical Council, USA

Dr C E Lumley, Associate Director, Centre for Medicines Research, UK

Ms V M Marshall, Director, Regulatory Affairs, Pfizer Central Research, UK

Dr M. Mitchell, Director, Astra Clinical Unit, UK

Dr N McAuslane, Project Manager, Centre for Medicines Research, UK

Professor C H Naito, Honorary Chairman, Department of Internal Medicine, Tokyo Teishin Hospital, Japan

Dr M Papaluca, Senior Medical Director, Pharmaceutical Division, Ministry of Health, Italy

Dr J Patterson, International Medical Director, Zeneca Pharmaceuticals, UK

Professor M D Rawlins, Chairman, Committee on Safety of Medicines, Professor of Clinical Pharmacology, University of Newcastle upon Tyne, UK

Professor J Schou, Chairman, Danish Committee on Adverse Drug Reactions, Institute of Pharmacology, Denmark

Dr W L Thompson, Chief Scientific Officer, Eli Lilly & Company, USA

Mr A Towse, Director, Office of Health Economics, UK

Dr K Voith, Bureau of Human Prescription Drugs, Health Protection Branch, Canada

Professor S R Walker, Director, Centre for Medicines Research, UK

Dr E C K Wong, Medical Director, Astra Asia Regional Office, Singapore

Dr A J J Wood, Professor of Pharmacology, Professor of Medicine, Department of Pharmacology, Vanderbilt University School of Medicine, USA

Index

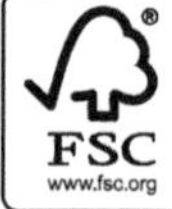 MIX
Papier aus verantwortungsvollen Quellen
Paper from responsible sources
FSC® C105338

If you have any concerns about our products,
you can contact us on
ProductSafety@springernature.com

In case Publisher is established outside the EU,
the EU authorized representative is:
**Springer Nature Customer Service Center GmbH
Europaplatz 3, 69115 Heidelberg, Germany**

Printed by Libri Plureos GmbH
in Hamburg, Germany